Frye's
3000
Nursing
Bullets

NCLEX-RN

FIFTH EDITION

Charles M. Frye, RN, MEd, JD

President
West Haven University
Salt Lake City, Utah

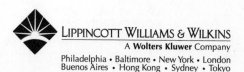

LIPPINCOTT WILLIAMS & WILKINS
A **Wolters Kluwer** Company

Philadelphia • Baltimore • New York • London
Buenos Aires • Hong Kong • Sydney • Tokyo

STAFF

Publisher
Judith A. Schilling McCann, RN, MSN

Editorial Director
William J. Kelly

Clinical Director
Joan M. Robinson, RN, MSN

Senior Art Director
Arlene Putterman

Senior Associate Editor
Elizabeth P. Lowe

Editor
Karla M. Schroeder

Clinical Editors
Beverly Tscheschlog, RN, BS
(clinical project manager);
Maryann Foley, RN, BSN;
Mary F. Gerard, RN, BSN, CCRN

Copy Editors
Kimberly Bilotta (supervisor),
Heather Ditch, Dona Hightower,
Irene Pontarelli, Dorothy P. Terry

Digital Composition Services
Diane Paluba (manager),
Joyce Rossi Biletz (senior desktop
assistant), Donna S. Morris (project
manager)

Manufacturing
Patricia K. Dorshaw (manager),
Beth Janae Orr (book production
manager)

Editorial Assistants
Megan Aldinger, Tara Carter-Bell,
Arlene C. Claffee, Linda Ruhf

Indexer
Barbara Hodgson

The clinical procedures described and recommended in this publication are based on research and consultation with nursing, medical, and legal authorities. To the best of our knowledge, these procedures reflect currently accepted practice; nevertheless, they can't be considered absolute and universal recommendations. For individual application, all recommendations must be considered in light of the patient's clinical condition and, before administration of new or infrequently used drugs, in light of the latest package-insert information. The authors and the publisher disclaim responsibility for any adverse effects resulting directly or indirectly from the suggested procedures, from any undetected errors, or from the reader's misunderstanding of the text.

FBRN010803–040706

Library of Congress
Cataloging-in-Publication Data

Frye, Charles M.
Frye's 3000 nursing bullets NCLEX-RN / Charles M. Frye.— 5th ed.
  p. ; cm.
  Rev. ed. of: Frye's 2,500 nursing bullets NCLEX-RN. 4th ed. 2000. Includes index.
  1. Nursing — Examinations, questions, etc. 2. Nursing — Outlines, syllabi, etc.
  [DNLM: 1. Nursing — Examination Questions. WY 18.2 F948f 2004] I. Title: Frye's three thousand nursing bullets NCLEX-RN. II. Title: 3000 nursing bullets NCLEX-RN. III. Frye, Charles M. Frye's 2,500 nursing bullets NCLEX-RN. IV. Title.
RT55.F793 2004
610.73'076—dc21
ISBN 1-58255-277-0 (pbk. : alk. paper)   2003012619

Contents

Contributors and consultants   v

Preface   vi

How to use this book   vii

Introduction   ix

3000 NURSING BULLETS ■ NCLEX-RN   1–226

Index   227

To my wonderful wife,
Lailani Tisbe-Frye, RN, BSN,
who has made all of my goals achievable
and every dream a reality.

Contributors and consultants

Elizabeth (Libby) A. Archer, RN, EdDc
Assistant Professor
Baptist College of Health Sciences
Memphis, Tenn.

Charlene K. Eshleman, RN, BSN, MSN
Clinical Nurse Specialist
Lancaster Regional Medical Center
Lancaster, Pa.

Mercy Flynn, RN
Coordinator, Instructor in Nursing
Christus Spohn Hospital, Coastal Bend College
Beeville, Tex.

Connie S. Heflin, RN, MSN
Professor of Nursing
Paducah Community Hospital
Paducah, Ky.

Shelton M. Hisley, RNC, PhD, WHNP
Assistant Professor of Nursing
The University of North Carolina at Wilmington

Gwendolyn L. Jordan, RN, MSN
Carolina College of Health Sciences
Charlotte, N.C.

Preface

I remember in great detail preparing to take the state licensing examination for registered nurses. Of all the memories I associate with that event, the most vivid is my frantic search through the bookstores for the "right" review book that would provide answers to the test. I didn't have the time and didn't want to spend all my waking hours reading one of those 500-page review books, but nothing else was available — until now.

This book is different from other review books you've seen or used. You're holding 3,000 nursing bullets — concise information that provides answers to questions not only on the upcoming NCLEX-RN, but also on the NCLEX-PN, Commission on Graduates of Foreign Nursing Schools (CGFNS) test, and any other nursing examination. How do these bullets work for you? They're concentrated nursing facts, stated in one or two sentences that are free of unnecessary or obscure words.

Test-question writers can create lengthy and time-consuming situations, provide minute (but not necessarily meaningful) details, and ask tricky questions that any of us can misunderstand. Even so, they can't change nursing facts. These 3,000 nursing bullets are just that — facts. They're the answers you need for test questions.

Passing the examination is a necessary step in the licensing process, and you must be prepared for it. This book can help you meet that challenge. Good luck.

How to use this book

Frye's 3000 Nursing Bullets NCLEX-RN, Fifth Edition, is designed to help you review for the NCLEX-RN effectively and efficiently. This book gives you nursing information for every clinical situation and setting — the very facts that question writers must draw on in devising the test.

Follow these suggestions to get the most from this unique book:

■ Read the introduction to prepare for computerized adaptive testing, learn about the NCLEX-RN test plan, and develop effective test-taking strategies.

■ Study the key facts as they're presented in random order. You'll realize two benefits from this approach: You'll master essential data in psychiatric, pediatric, maternal, and medical-surgical nursing as well as the important concepts in nursing fundamentals and you'll prepare yourself for the computerized NCLEX-RN, which also presents questions in a random style. (Note: After each bulleted fact in this book, the applicable clinical topic area appears in parentheses: FND for fundamentals, MAT for maternal-neonatal nursing, M-S for medical-surgical nursing, PED for pediatric nursing, and PSY for psychiatric nursing.)

■ Review groups of nursing bullets throughout the day. Because this book is compact and easy to carry, you can take it with you wherever you go and review a few bullets whenever you have a spare minute — while waiting for class to begin, during a break between labs, or while riding the bus or train.

■ Use the book to create questions to quiz your study partner or members of your study group.

No matter how you choose to use this versatile book, you'll find that each nursing bullet is brief, easy to read, and free from distracting clinical situations and excess wording. You'll find that you'll easily remember and identify the facts, no matter what form they take on the test. Because each bullet has been reviewed by a clinical expert, you can be sure that all the information is up-to-date and clinically accurate.

You've spent years studying to become a nurse and months preparing for the NCLEX-RN. Now, with *Frye's 3000 Nursing Bullets NCLEX-RN*, Fifth Edition, you can take the last step to licensure with confidence.

Introduction

In the United States, if you want to work as a registered nurse, you need a license from the nursing licensure authority in the state where you plan to practice. To get a license, you need to pass the National Council Licensure Examination for Registered Nurses (NCLEX-RN). This book will help you do just that. Its 3,000 bullets of nursing facts will expand and reinforce your nursing knowledge base. This introduction will prepare you for the examination by describing computerized adaptive testing, explaining the NCLEX-RN test plan, and providing effective test-taking strategies.

Scheduling your test
To schedule your NCLEX-RN, apply to your state board of nursing for testing. When your application is approved, the Educational Testing Service Data Center will send you an Authorization to Test and will advise you to make an examination appointment at one of the Pearson Professional Centers throughout the country.

When scheduling your NCLEX-RN, remember that the test takes up to 5 hours and is offered 15 hours daily, Monday through Saturday, and sometimes on Sunday. The Pearson Professional Center will schedule you for testing within 30 days of your call (or within 45 days for retesting). If you need to reschedule your examination appointment, call the Pearson Professional Center at least 3 days beforehand.

Understanding computerized adaptive testing
Since April of 1994, the NCLEX-RN has been a computerized test. It requires you to answer a sufficient number of questions of various levels of difficulty to demonstrate minimum competence as an entry-level nurse. It's adaptive because it selects harder or easier questions based on your response to previous questions. For example, if you answer a medium-level question correctly, the computer will pose a more difficult question next. If you answer incorrectly, it will choose an easier one.

The test bank includes thousands of questions categorized by level of difficulty and the NCLEX-RN test plan. From this bank, the computer continues to pull questions until you demonstrate competence in all parts of the test plan. Therefore, each test is different and may require 75 to 265 questions to complete.

Before the test, a proctor will help you get started at a computer terminal. The test will begin with brief instructions and a practice session of 15 questions. During the practice session and the test, use the mouse to move the cursor to the four answer options and to select your answer. To avoid unintentional answers, the computer will ask you to confirm your answer selection.

During the test, the computer will display one question at a time. If a case study is included, it will appear to the left of the question. Consider each question carefully. Then use the mouse to move to the option that best answers the question. Because the computer doesn't let you skip questions or return to previous items, you must answer every question until the test ends. The testing period includes a mandatory 10-minute break after 2 hours and an optional break 90 minutes after testing resumes.

Understanding the NCLEX-RN test plan

The NCLEX-RN test plan classifies questions by the five steps of the nursing process and the four categories of client needs. Each test question reflects one nursing process step and one client needs category.

Nursing process steps

The nursing process is a five-step method of performing nursing care. On the NCLEX-RN test, each nursing process step carries equal weight and accounts for 20% of the test questions.

- *Assessment* refers to forming a database by gathering subjective and objective information about a patient.

- *Analysis,* or nursing diagnosis, refers to identifying actual or potential problems based on assessment findings.

- *Planning* refers to establishing goals to meet the patient's needs and developing strategies for achieving those goals.

- *Implementation* refers to putting the nursing care plan into action and performing actions that enable the patient to achieve the goals.

- *Evaluation* refers to measuring the extent of goal achievement.

Client needs categories

Client needs categories are based on data from a major nursing job survey. These client needs are further divided into subcategories that define the content contained within each of the four major client needs categories. Each subcategory accounts for a varying percentage of the test questions.

- Safe, effective care environment refers to promoting environmental safety, providing effective care, ensuring quality, and performing treatments and procedures safely and effectively. Subcategories include:
  - Management of care (7% to 13% of the test)
  - Safety and infection control (5% to 11% of the test).

- Health promotion and maintenance refers to meeting the patient's needs by promoting growth and development, self-care, support system integrity, and disease prevention and early treatment. Subcategories include:
  - Growth and development through the life span (7% to 13% of the test)
  - Prevention and early detection of disease (5% to 11% of the test).

- Psychosocial integrity refers to meeting the patient's psychosocial needs during times of stress or crisis by promoting coping skills and adaptation throughout the life cycle. Subcategories include:
  - Coping and adaptation (5% to 11% of the test)
  - Psychosocial adaptation (5% to 11% of the test).

- Physiological integrity refers to meeting the physiological needs of a patient with a life-threatening or recurring condition (or one at risk for complications or adverse effects of treatments) by providing care, reducing risks, and promoting physiological adaptation and comfort. Subcategories include:
  - Basic care and comfort (7% to 13% of the test)
  - Pharmacological and parenteral therapies (5% to 11% of the test)
  - Reduction of risk potential (12% to 18% of the test)
  - Physiological adaptation (12% to 18% of the test).

Studying for the examination

To study for the NCLEX-RN as effectively as possible and enhance your ability to retain pertinent information, follow these study tips:

- Familiarize yourself with all examination topics.

- Answer as many practice questions as possible. (You may want to use this book's bullets to develop questions with a study partner.)

- Understand the parts of a test question. On the NCLEX-RN, each multiple-choice question has a stem (the question itself) and four options: a key (correct answer) and three distracters (incorrect answers). A brief case study may precede any question. New alternative item format questions may also include multiple-choice items in which there may be more than one correct response, fill in the blank, or items asking a candidate to identify an area on a picture or graphic. Any item formats may include tables, charts, or graphic images. If you're well versed in nursing, the format of the question shouldn't present a problem.

- Use additional study guides as resources, such as the American Nursing Review for NCLEX-RN, if desired.

- Organize a study group with other nursing students or take an NCLEX review course.

- Ask a colleague or nursing instructor to clarify unfamiliar or complex material.

Planning for the examination

Remember that the NCLEX-RN poses certain physical demands. To cope with these demands, ensure your best test performance, and help you plan for the examination, use these pointers:

- Schedule your test appointment at a testing center near your home, if possible. Before the test, assess the parking facilities and determine travel time.

- Make reservations well in advance at a hotel near the testing center if you must travel a long distance.

- Schedule your test appointment to take advantage of your peak-performance time.

- Avoid late-night, last-minute cramming. Obtain sufficient sleep the night before the test.

- Eat a well-balanced meal before the test.

- Wear layers of clothes that can be removed, as needed, to keep you comfortable.

- Take your Authorization to Test and two forms of identification with signatures (including one photographic identification) to the testing center. You can't take the examination without them.

■ Use simple relaxation techniques, such as progressive relaxation, during the test to reduce anxiety.

■ Take a strategic break.

Developing test-taking skills

Knowing the facts isn't all you need to pass the NCLEX-RN. You also need to know how to take the test. To sharpen your test-taking skills, review these guidelines:

■ Check case studies closely for information needed to answer the question correctly.

■ Look for clue words, such as *best, first, most,* and *not,* in the question's stem. These words, which may be highlighted, aid in selecting the correct answer.

■ Imagine the correct response when reading the stem. If it appears as one of the four options, it's probably the correct one.

■ Read every question — and all four of its options — carefully before making your final selection.

■ Reread the stem and options when two options seem equally correct; look again for clues or differences that can help you select the correct answer. When in doubt, make an educated guess. Remember: You can't skip questions.

■ Don't panic if a question covers an unfamiliar topic. Draw on your knowledge of similar problems and nursing principles to help eliminate options and increase the chance of choosing the correct answer.

■ Take your time and pace yourself. Don't spend excessive time on any one question.

■ Don't be distracted by other candidates or the apparent length of their tests. Keep in mind that each test is individualized.

■ Use break periods to rest your mind and body — for example, eat a small snack, stretch, or do relaxation exercises.

A note to foreign nurse graduates

If you were educated in a foreign country, you must meet the requirements for foreign nurse graduates set by the state board of nursing in the state where you plan to practice. Most states require a certificate from the Commission on Graduates of Foreign Nursing Schools (CGFNS) before you take the NCLEX-RN.

Eligibility requirements for the CGFNS examination include successful completion of a secondary education; a valid, current nursing license in the country in which you were educated; and graduation from a well-balanced, 2-year (or longer) nursing education program in a government-approved school.

The CGFNS examination tests your nursing knowledge and English proficiency. Its nursing portion follows the NCLEX-RN test plan and reliably predicts success on NCLEX-RN. Its English portion consists of written and listening sections. Its results reach you by mail 8 to 10 weeks after the test; passage of the test earns you a CGFNS certificate.

You can get application forms and the *CGFNS Guidebook for Applicants* through U.S. embassies in foreign countries, national nurses' associations, and CGFNS at 3600 Market Street, Philadelphia, PA 19104-2651. The *Guidebook for Applicants* presents eligibility requirements, application procedures, fees, and suggestions for CGFNS test preparation.

Frye's

3000

Nursing
Bullets

NCLEX-RN

FIFTH EDITION

A child in Bryant's traction who is younger than age 3 or weighs less than 30 lb (13.6 kg) should have the buttocks slightly elevated and clear of the bed. The knees should be slightly flexed, and the legs should be extended at a right angle to the body. The body provides the traction mechanism. **(PED)**

Unlike false labor, true labor produces regular rhythmic contractions, abdominal discomfort, progressive descent of the fetus, bloody show, and progressive effacement and dilation of the cervix. **(MAT)**

Pernicious anemia results from the failure to absorb vitamin B_{12} in the GI tract and causes primarily GI and neurologic signs and symptoms. **(M-S)**

In a patient with hypokalemia (serum potassium level below 3.5 mEq/L), presenting signs and symptoms include muscle weakness and cardiac arrhythmias. **(M-S)**

According to Kübler-Ross, the five stages of death and dying are denial, anger, bargaining, depression, and acceptance. **(PSY)**

During cardiac arrest, if an I.V. route is unavailable, epinephrine can be administered endotracheally. **(M-S)**

To help a mother break the suction of her breast-feeding infant, the nurse should teach her to insert a finger at the corner of the infant's mouth. **(MAT)**

A patient who has a pressure ulcer should consume a high-protein, high-calorie diet, unless contraindicated. **(M-S)**

The CK-MB isoenzyme level is used to assess tissue damage in myocardial infarction. **(M-S)**

After a 12-hour fast, the normal fasting blood glucose level is 80 to 120 mg/dl. **(M-S)**

A blood pressure cuff that's too narrow can cause a falsely elevated blood pressure reading. **(FND)**

A blood pressure cuff that's too wide can cause a falsely decreased blood pressure reading. **(FND)**

A patient who is experiencing digoxin toxicity may report nausea, vomiting, diplopia, blurred vision, light flashes, and yellow-green halos around images. **(M-S)**

- Administering high levels of oxygen to a premature neonate can cause blindness as a result of retrolental fibroplasia. **(MAT)**

- When preparing a single injection for a patient who takes regular and neutral protein Hagedorn insulin, the nurse should draw the regular insulin into the syringe first so that it does not contaminate the regular insulin. **(FND)**

- *Anuria* is daily urine output of less than 100 ml. **(M-S)**

- In remittent fever, the body temperature varies over a 24-hour period, but remains elevated. **(M-S)**

- *Rhonchi* are the rumbling sounds heard on lung auscultation. They are more pronounced during expiration than during inspiration. **(FND)**

- *Gavage* is forced feeding, usually through a gastric tube (a tube passed into the stomach through the mouth). **(FND)**

- Risk of a fat embolism is greatest in the first 48 hours after the fracture of a long bone. It's manifested by respiratory distress. **(M-S)**

- To help venous blood return in a patient who is in shock, the nurse should elevate the patient's legs no more than 45 degrees. This procedure is contraindicated in a patient with a head injury. **(M-S)**

- According to Maslow's hierarchy of needs, physiologic needs (air, water, food, shelter, sex, activity, and comfort) have the highest priority. **(FND)**

- The safest and surest way to verify a patient's identity is to check the identification band on his wrist. **(FND)**

- In the therapeutic environment, the patient's safety is the primary concern. **(FND)**

- The pulse deficit is the difference between the apical and radial pulse rates, when taken simultaneously by two nurses. **(M-S)**

- To reduce the patient's risk of vomiting and aspiration, the nurse should schedule postural drainage before meals or 2 to 4 hours after meals. **(M-S)**

- Blood pressure can be measured directly by intra-arterial insertion of a catheter connected to a pressure-monitoring device. **(M-S)**

■ A positive Kernig's sign, seen in meningitis, occurs when an attempt to flex the hip of a recumbent patient causes painful spasms of the hamstring muscle and resistance to further extension of the leg at the knee. (M-S)

■ In a patient with a fractured, dislocated femur, treatment begins with reduction and immobilization of the affected leg. (M-S)

■ Herniated nucleus pulposus (intervertebral disk) most commonly occurs in the lumbar and lumbosacral regions. (M-S)

■ *Laminectomy* is surgical removal of the herniated portion of an intervertebral disk. (M-S)

■ Surgical treatment of a gastric ulcer includes severing the vagus nerve (vagotomy) to reduce the amount of gastric acid secreted by the gastric cells. (M-S)

■ *Flight of ideas* is an alteration in thought processes that's characterized by skipping from one topic to another, unrelated topic. (PSY)

■ *La belle indifférence* is the lack of concern for a profound disability, such as blindness or paralysis that may occur in a patient who has a conversion disorder. (PSY)

■ In an infant, a bulging fontanel is the most significant sign of increasing intracranial pressure. (PED)

■ Moderate anxiety decreases a person's ability to perceive and concentrate. The person is selectively inattentive (focuses on immediate concerns), and the perceptual field narrows. (PSY)

■ A patient who has a phobic disorder uses self-protective avoidance as an ego defense mechanism. (PSY)

■ In a patient who has anorexia nervosa, the highest treatment priority is correction of nutritional and electrolyte imbalances. (PSY)

■ A patient who is taking lithium must undergo regular (usually once a month) monitoring of the blood lithium level because the margin between therapeutic and toxic levels is narrow. A normal laboratory value is 0.5 to 1.5 mEq/L. (PSY)

■ *Valsalva's maneuver* is forced exhalation against a closed glottis, as when taking a deep breath, blowing air out, or bearing down. (M-S)

■ Early signs and symptoms of alcohol withdrawal include anxiety, anorexia, tremors, and insomnia. They may begin up to 8 hours after the last alcohol intake. **(PSY)**

■ Al-Anon is a support group for families of alcoholics. **(PSY)**

■ The nurse shouldn't administer chlorpromazine (Thorazine) to a patient who has ingested alcohol because it may cause oversedation and respiratory depression. **(PSY)**

■ When mean arterial pressure falls below 60 mm Hg and systolic blood pressure falls below 80 mm Hg, vital organ perfusion is seriously compromised. **(M-S)**

■ Lidocaine (Xylocaine) is the drug of choice for reducing premature ventricular contractions. **(M-S)**

■ Lithium toxicity can occur when sodium and fluid intake are insufficient, causing lithium retention. **(PSY)**

■ *Amniotomy* is artificial rupture of the amniotic membranes. **(MAT)**

■ An alcoholic who achieves sobriety is called a *recovering alcoholic* because no cure for alcoholism exists. **(PSY)**

■ A patient is at greatest risk of dying during the first 24 to 48 hours after a myocardial infarction. **(M-S)**

■ During a myocardial infarction, the left ventricle usually sustains the greatest damage. **(M-S)**

■ The pain of a myocardial infarction results from myocardial ischemia caused by anoxia. **(M-S)**

■ For a patient in cardiac arrest, the first priority is to establish an airway. **(M-S)**

■ The universal sign for choking is clutching the hand to the throat. **(M-S)**

■ For a patient who has heart failure or cardiogenic pulmonary edema, nursing interventions focus on decreasing venous return to the heart and increasing left ventricular output. These interventions include placing the patient in high Fowler's position and administering oxygen, diuretics, and positive inotropic drugs as prescribed. **(M-S)**

A positive tuberculin skin test is an induration of 10 mm or greater at the injection site.   (M-S)

The signs and symptoms of histoplasmosis, a chronic systemic fungal infection, resemble those of tuberculosis.   (M-S)

Fluid oscillation in the tubing of a chest drainage system indicates that the system is working properly.   (FND)

In burn victims, the leading cause of death is respiratory compromise. The second leading cause is infection.   (M-S)

The exocrine function of the pancreas is the secretion of enzymes used to digest carbohydrates, fats, and proteins.   (M-S)

A patient who has hepatitis A (infectious hepatitis) should consume a diet that's moderately high in fat and high in carbohydrate and protein, and should eat the largest meal in the morning.   (M-S)

The nurse should place a patient who has a Sengstaken-Blakemore tube in semi-Fowler position.   (FND)

Esophageal balloon tamponade shouldn't be inflated greater than 20 mm Hg.   (M-S)

Overproduction of prolactin by the pituitary gland can cause galactorrhea (excessive or abnormal lactation) and amenorrhea (absence of menstruation).   (M-S)

Intermittent claudication (pain during ambulation or other movement that's relieved with rest) is a classic symptom of arterial insufficiency in the leg.   (M-S)

During pregnancy, weight gain averages 25 to 30 lb (11 to 13.5 kg).
                                                                       (MAT)

In bladder carcinoma, the most common finding is gross, painless hematuria.   (M-S)

The nurse can elicit Trousseau's sign by occluding the brachial or radial artery. Hand and finger spasms that occur during occlusion indicate Trousseau's sign and suggest hypocalcemia.   (FND)

Parenteral administration of heparin sodium is contraindicated in patients with renal or liver disease, GI bleeding, or recent surgery or trauma; in pregnant patients; and in women older than age 60.   (M-S)

■ Drugs that potentiate the effects of anticoagulants include aspirin, chloral hydrate, glucagon, anabolic steroids, and chloramphenicol.   **(M-S)**

■ According to Erikson, the school-age child (ages 6 to 12) is in the industry-versus-inferiority stage of psychosocial development.   **(PSY)**

■ For a burn patient, care priorities include maintaining a patent airway, preventing or correcting fluid and electrolyte imbalances, controlling pain, and preventing infection.   **(M-S)**

■ Elastic stockings should be worn on both legs.   **(M-S)**

■ *Active immunization* is the formation of antibodies within the body in response to vaccination or exposure to disease.   **(M-S)**

■ *Passive immunization* is administration of antibodies that were preformed outside the body.   **(M-S)**

■ Chickenpox causes a rash that has four stages: macules, papules, vesicles, and crusts. Lesions of various stages occur simultaneously during the illness.   **(PED)**

■ Rubella has a teratogenic effect on the fetus during the first trimester. It produces abnormalities in up to 40% of cases without interrupting the pregnancy.   **(MAT)**

■ To calculate a pediatric dose using Clark's rule, the nurse should multiply the adult dose by the child's weight in pounds and divide the result by 150.   **(PED)**

■ To calculate a pediatric dose using Young's rule, the nurse should multiply the adult dose by the child's age in years and divide the result by the sum of the child's age plus 12.   **(PED)**

■ A patient who is receiving digoxin (Lanoxin) shouldn't receive a calcium preparation because of the increased risk of digoxin toxicity. Concomitant use may affect cardiac contractility and lead to arrhythmias.   **(M-S)**

■ For blood transfusion in an adult, the appropriate needle size is 16 to 20G.   **(FND)**

■ *Intermittent positive-pressure breathing* is inflation of the lung during inspiration with compressed air or oxygen. The goal of this inflation is to keep the lung open.   **(M-S)**

To prevent infection in patients with sickle cell anemia, penicillin prophylaxis is started at age 2 months. **(PED)**

Wristdrop is caused by paralysis of the extensor muscles in the forearm and hand. **(M-S)**

Footdrop results from excessive plantar flexion and is usually a complication of prolonged bed rest. **(M-S)**

A patient who has gonorrhea may be treated with penicillin and probenecid (Benemid). Probenecid delays the excretion of penicillin and keeps this antibiotic in the body longer. **(M-S)**

Intractable pain is pain that incapacitates a patient and can't be relieved by drugs. **(IND)**

In an emergency, consent for treatment can be obtained by fax, telephone, or other telegraphic means. **(FND)**

In patients who have glucose-6-phosphate dehydrogenase (G6PD) deficiency, the red blood cells can't metabolize adequate amounts of glucose, and hemolysis occurs. **(M-S)**

Decibel is the unit of measurement of sound. **(FND)**

On-call medication is medication that should be ready for immediate administration when the call to administer it's received. **(M-S)**

If gagging, nausea, or vomiting occurs when an airway is removed, the nurse should place the patient in a lateral position with the upper arm supported on a pillow. **(M-S)**

Emancipated minors are individuals younger than the age of majority (usually age 18 or 21) who aren't under parental control, such as married minors, those who serve in the military, and college students who live away from home. **(PED)**

Informed consent is required for any invasive procedure. **(FND)**

A patient who can't write his name to give consent for treatment must make an X in the presence of two witnesses, such as a nurse, priest, or physician. **(FND)**

When a postoperative patient arrives in the recovery room, the nurse should position the patient on his side or with his head turned to the side and the chin extended. **(M-S)**

In the immediate postoperative period, the nurse should report a respiratory rate greater than 30, temperature greater than 100° F (37.8° C) or below 97° F (36.1° C), or a significant drop in blood pressure or rise in pulse rate from the baseline.   (M-S)

Immunity to rubella can be measured by a hemagglutination inhibition test (rubella titer). This test identifies exposure to rubella infection and determines susceptibility in pregnant women. In a woman, a titer greater than 1:8 indicates immunity.   (MAT)

When used to describe the degree of fetal descent during labor, *floating* means the presenting part isn't engaged in the pelvic inlet, but is freely movable (ballotable) above the pelvic inlet.   (MAT)

Irreversible brain damage may occur if the central nervous system is deprived of oxygen for more than 4 minutes.   (M-S)

When used to describe the degree of fetal descent, *engagement* means when the largest diameter of the presenting part has passed through the pelvic inlet.   (MAT)

The Z-track I.M. injection technique seals the drug deep into the muscle, thereby minimizing skin irritation and staining. It requires a needle that's 1″ (2.5 cm) or longer.   (FND)

Fetal station indicates the location of the presenting part in relation to the ischial spine. It's described as –1, –2, –3, –4, or –5 to indicate the number of centimeters above the level of the ischial spine; station –5 is at the pelvic inlet.   (MAT)

Fetal station also is described as +1, +2, +3, +4, or +5 to indicate the number of centimeters it is below the level of the ischial spine; station 0 is at the level of the ischial spine.   (MAT)

During the first stage of labor, the side-lying position usually provides the greatest degree of comfort, although the patient may assume any comfortable position.   (MAT)

During delivery, if the umbilical cord can't be loosened and slipped from around the neonate's neck, it should be clamped with two clamps and cut between the clamps.   (MAT)

An Apgar score of 7 to 10 indicates no immediate distress, 4 to 6 indicates moderate distress, and 0 to 3 indicates severe distress.   (MAT)

Treatment for polycythemia vera includes administering oxygen, radio-isotope therapy, or chemotherapy agents, such as chlorambucil and nitrogen mustard, to suppress bone marrow growth.   (M-S)

A patient with acute renal failure should receive a high-calorie diet that's low in protein as well as potassium and sodium.   (M-S)

Addison's disease is caused by hypofunction of the adrenal gland and is characterized by fatigue, anemia, weight loss, and bronze skin pigmentation. Without cortisol replacement therapy, it's usually fatal.   (M-S)

In the event of fire, the acronym most often used is RACE. (R) Remove the patient. (A) Activate the alarm. (C) Attempt to contain the fire by closing the door. (E) Extinguish the fire if it can be done safely.   (FND)

When caring for a depressed patient, the nurse's first priority is safety because of the increased risk of suicide.   (PSY)

Glaucoma is managed conservatively with beta-adrenergic blockers such as timolol (Timoptic), which decrease sympathetic impulses to the eye, and with miotic eyedrops such as pilocarpine (Isopto Carpine), which constrict the pupils.   (M-S)

Miotics effectively treat glaucoma by reducing intraocular pressure. They do this by constricting the pupil, contracting the ciliary muscles, opening the anterior chamber angle, and increasing the outflow of aqueous humor.   (M-S)

While a patient is receiving heparin, the nurse should monitor the partial thromboplastin time.   (M-S)

Urinary frequency, incontinence, or both can occur after catheter removal. Incontinence may be manifested as dribbling.   (M-S)

When teaching a patient about colostomy care, the nurse should instruct the patient to hang the irrigation reservoir 18" to 22" (45 to 55 cm) above the stoma, insert the catheter 2" to 4" (5 to 10 cm) into the stoma, irrigate the stoma with 17 to 34 oz (503 to 1,005 ml) of water at a temperature of 105° to 110° F (40° to 43° C) once a day, clean the area around the stoma with soap and water before applying a new bag, and use a protective skin covering, such as a Stomahesive wafer, karaya paste, or karaya ring, around the stoma.   (M-S)

■ The first sign of Hodgkin's disease is painless, superficial lymphade-nopathy, typically found under one arm or on one side of the neck in the cervical chain. **(M-S)**

■ A registered nurse should assign a licensed vocational nurse or licensed practical nurse to perform bedside care, such as suctioning and drug administration. **(FND)**

■ To differentiate true cyanosis from deposition of certain pigments, the nurse should press the skin over the discolored area. Cyanotic skin blanches, but pigmented skin doesn't. **(M-S)**

■ A patient who has a gastric ulcer is most likely to report pain during or shortly after eating. **(M-S)**

■ Widening pulse pressure is a sign of increasing intracranial pressure. For example, the blood pressure may rise from 120/80 to 160/60 mm Hg. **(M-S)**

■ In a burn victim, a primary goal of wound care is to prevent contamina-tion by microorganisms. **(M-S)**

■ To prevent external rotation in a patient who has had hip nailing, the nurse places trochanter rolls from the knee to the ankle of the affected leg. **(M-S)**

■ Severe hip pain after the insertion of a hip prosthesis indicates dislodg-ment. If this occurs, before calling the physician, the nurse should assess the patient for shortening of the leg, external rotation, and absence of reflexes. **(M-S)**

■ To elicit Moro's reflex, the nurse holds the neonate in both hands and suddenly, but gently, drops the neonate's head backward. Normally, the neonate abducts and extends all extremities bilaterally and symmetri-cally, forms a C shape with the thumb and forefinger, and first adducts and then flexes the extremities. **(MAT)**

■ *Echolalia* is parrotlike repetition of another person's words or phrases. **(PSY)**

■ According to psychoanalytic theory, the ego is the part of the psyche that controls internal demands and interacts with the outside world at the conscious, preconscious, and unconscious levels. **(PSY)**

▇ According to psychoanalytic theory, the superego is the part of the psyche that's composed of morals, values, and ethics. It continually evaluates thoughts and actions, rewarding the good and punishing the bad. (Think of the superego as the "supercop" of the unconscious.)   (PSY)

▇ According to psychoanalytic theory, the id is the part of the psyche that contains instinctual drives. (Remember *i* for instinctual and *d* for drive.)
(PSY)

▇ According to Erikson, from birth to age 12 months, the child is in the trust-versus-mistrust stage of psychosocial development.   (PED)

▇ Pregnancy-induced hypertension (preeclampsia) is an increase in blood pressure of 30/15 mm Hg over baseline or blood pressure of 140/95 mm Hg on two occasions at least 6 hours apart accompanied by edema and albuminuria after 20 weeks' gestation.   (MAT)

▇ Positive signs of pregnancy include ultrasound evidence, fetal heart tones, and fetal movement felt by the examiner (not usually present until 4 months' gestation).   (MAT)

▇ *Goodell's sign* is softening of the cervix.   (MAT)

▇ *Hegar's sign* is softening of the lower segment of the uterus.   (MAT)

▇ Quickening, a presumptive sign of pregnancy, occurs between 16 and 19 weeks' gestation.   (MAT)

▇ Ovulation ceases during pregnancy.   (MAT)

▇ Any vaginal bleeding during pregnancy should be considered a complication until proven otherwise.   (MAT)

▇ To estimate the date of delivery using Nägele's rule, the nurse counts backward 3 months from the first day of the last menstrual period and then adds 7 days to this date.   (MAT)

▇ At 12 weeks' gestation, the fundus should be at the top of the symphysis pubis.   (MAT)

▇ *Koplik's spots* are small, irregular, red spots with minute, bluish white centers that appear on the buccal mucosa of patients with measles (rubeola).
(PED)

▇ As much as 75% of renal function is lost before blood urea nitrogen and serum creatinine levels rise above normal.   (M-S)

■ When compensatory efforts are present in acid-base balance, partial pressure of arterial carbon dioxide ($Paco_2$) and bicarbonate (HCO_3^-) always point in the same direction:

pH↓ $Paco_2$↑ HCO_3^-↑ = respiratory acidosis compensated

pH↑ $Paco_2$↓ HCO_3^-↓ = respiratory alkalosis compensated

pH↓ $Paco_2$↓ HCO_3^-↓ = metabolic acidosis compensated

pH↑ $Paco_2$↑ HCO_3^-↑ = metabolic alkalosis compensated.   (M-S)

■ *Polyuria* is urine output of 2,500 ml or more within 24 hours.   (M-S)

■ The presenting sign of pleuritis is chest pain that is usually unilateral and related to respiratory movement.   (M-S)

■ If a patient can't void, the first nursing action should be bladder palpation to assess for bladder distention.   (FND)

■ If a patient has a gastric drainage tube in place, the nurse should expect the physician to order potassium chloride.   (M-S)

■ Cow's milk shouldn't be given to infants younger than age 1 because it has a low linoleic acid content and its protein is difficult for infants to digest.   (MAT)

■ An increased pulse rate is one of the first indications of respiratory difficulty. It occurs because the heart attempts to compensate for a decreased oxygen supply to the tissues by pumping more blood.   (M-S)

■ If jaundice is suspected in a neonate, the nurse should examine the infant under natural window light. If natural light is unavailable, the nurse should examine the infant under a white light.   (MAT)

■ *Denial* is the defense mechanism used by a patient who denies the reality of an event.   (PSY)

■ The three phases of a uterine contraction are increment, acme, and decrement.   (MAT)

■ The patient who uses a cane should carry it on the unaffected side and advance it at the same time as the affected extremity.   (FND)

■ To fit a supine patient for crutches, the nurse should measure from the axilla to the sole and add 2″ (5 cm) to that measurement.   (FND)

The intensity of a labor contraction can be assessed by the indentability of the uterine wall at the contraction's peak. Intensity is graded as mild (uterine muscle is somewhat tense), moderate (uterine muscle is moderately tense), or strong (uterine muscle is boardlike).   (MAT)

Chloasma, the mask of pregnancy, is pigmentation of a circumscribed area of skin (usually over the bridge of the nose and cheeks) that occurs in some pregnant women.   (MAT)

The gynecoid pelvis is most ideal for delivery. Other types include platypelloid (flat), anthropoid (apelike), and android (malelike).   (MAT)

Pregnant women should be advised that there is no safe level of alcohol intake.   (MAT)

In an adult, a hemoglobin level below 11 mg/dl suggests iron deficiency anemia and the need for further evaluation.   (M-S)

The normal partial pressure of oxygen in arterial blood is 95 mm Hg (plus or minus 5 mm Hg).   (M-S)

Vitamin C deficiency is characterized by brittle bones, pinpoint peripheral hemorrhages, and friable gums with loosened teeth.   (M-S)

Clinical manifestations of pulmonary embolism are variable, but increased respiratory rate, tachycardia, and hemoptysis are common.   (M-S)

In a psychiatric setting, seclusion is used to reduce overwhelming environmental stimulation, protect the patient from self-injury or injury to others, and prevent damage to hospital property. It's used for patients who don't respond to less restrictive interventions. Seclusion controls external behavior until the patient can assume self-control and helps the patient to regain self-control.   (PSY)

Tyramine-rich food, such as aged cheese, chicken liver, avocados, bananas, meat tenderizer, salami, bologna, Chianti wine, and beer may cause severe hypertension in a patient who takes a monoamine oxidase inhibitor.   (PSY)

A patient who takes a monoamine oxidase inhibitor should be weighed biweekly and monitored for suicidal tendencies.   (PSY)

If the patient who takes a monoamine oxidase inhibitor has palpitations, headaches, or severe orthostatic hypotension, the nurse should withhold the drug and notify the physician.   (PSY)

Normally, intraocular pressure is 12 to 20 mm Hg. It can be measured with a Schiøtz tonometer. **(M-S)**

The frequency of uterine contractions, which is measured in minutes, is the time from the beginning of one contraction to the beginning of the next. **(MAT)**

In early hemorrhagic shock, blood pressure may be normal, but respiratory and pulse rates are rapid. The patient may report thirst and may have clammy skin and piloerection (goose bumps). **(M-S)**

Assessment begins with the nurse's first encounter with the patient and continues throughout the patient's stay. The nurse obtains assessment data through the health history, physical examination, and review of diagnostic studies. **(FND)**

Cool, moist, pale skin, as occurs in shock, results from diversion of blood from the skin to the major organs. **(M-S)**

To assess capillary refill, the nurse applies pressure over the nail bed until blanching occurs, quickly releases the pressure, and notes the rate at which blanching fades. Capillary refill indicates perfusion, which decreases in shock, thereby lengthening refill time. Normal capillary refill is less than 3 seconds. **(M-S)**

Except for patients with renal failure, urine output of less than 30 ml/hour signifies dehydration and the potential for shock. **(M-S)**

The appropriate needle size for insulin injection is 25G and $5/8''$ long. **(FND)**

Residual urine is urine that remains in the bladder after voiding. The amount of residual urine is normally 50 to 100 ml. **(FND)**

In elderly patients, the most common fracture is hip fracture. Osteoporosis weakens the bones, predisposing these patients to fracture, which usually results from a fall. **(M-S)**

The five stages of the nursing process are assessment, nursing diagnosis, planning, implementation, and evaluation. **(FND)**

Assessment is the stage of the nursing process in which the nurse continuously collects data to identify a patient's actual and potential health needs. **(FND)**

Nursing diagnosis is the stage of the nursing process in which the nurse makes a clinical judgment about individual, family, or community responses to actual or potential health problems or life processes. **(FND)**

Planning is the stage of the nursing process in which the nurse assigns priorities to nursing diagnoses, defines short-term and long-term goals and expected outcomes, and establishes the nursing care plan. **(FND)**

Implementation is the stage of the nursing process in which the nurse puts the nursing care plan into action, delegates specific nursing interventions to members of the nursing team, and charts patient responses to nursing interventions. **(FND)**

Evaluation is the stage of the nursing process in which the nurse compares objective and subjective data with the outcome criteria and, if needed, modifies the nursing care plan. **(FND)**

Before angiography, the nurse should ask the patient whether he's allergic to the dye, shellfish, or iodine and advise him to take nothing by mouth for 8 hours before the procedure. **(M-S)**

During myelography, approximately 10 to 15 ml of cerebrospinal fluid is removed for laboratory studies and an equal amount of contrast media is injected. **(M-S)**

Vitamin K is administered to neonates to prevent hemorrhagic disorders because a neonate's intestine can't synthesize vitamin K. **(MAT)**

After angiography, the puncture site is covered with a pressure dressing and the affected part is immobilized for 8 hours to decrease the risk of bleeding. **(M-S)**

If a water-based medium was used during myelography, the patient remains on bed rest for 6 to 8 hours, with the head of the bed elevated 30 to 45 degrees. If an oil-based medium was used, the patient remains flat in bed for 6 to 24 hours. **(M-S)**

The level of amputation is determined by estimating the maximum viable tissue (tissue with adequate circulation) needed to develop a functional stump. **(M-S)**

Before internal fetal monitoring can be performed, a pregnant patient's cervix must be dilated at least 2 cm, the amniotic membranes must be ruptured, and the fetus's presenting part (scalp or buttocks) must be at station –1 or lower, so that a small electrode can be attached. **(MAT)**

■ Fetal alcohol syndrome presents in the first 24 hours after birth and produces lethargy, seizures, poor sucking reflex, abdominal distention, and respiratory difficulty. **(MAT)**

■ *Variability* is any change in the fetal heart rate (FHR) from its normal rate of 120 to 160 beats/minute. *Acceleration* is increased FHR; *deceleration* is decreased FHR. **(MAT)**

■ Heparin sodium is included in the dialysate used for renal dialysis. **(M-S)**

■ In a neonate, the symptoms of heroin withdrawal may begin several hours to 4 days after birth. **(MAT)**

■ In a neonate, the symptoms of methadone withdrawal may begin 7 days to several weeks after birth. **(MAT)**

■ In a neonate, the cardinal signs of narcotic withdrawal include coarse, flapping tremors; sleepiness; restlessness; prolonged, persistent, high-pitched cry; and irritability. **(MAT)**

■ The nurse should count a neonate's respirations for 1 full minute. **(MAT)**

■ Paroxysmal nocturnal dyspnea may indicate heart failure. **(M-S)**

■ A patient who takes a cardiac glycoside, such as digoxin, should consume a diet that includes high-potassium foods. **(M-S)**

■ The nurse should limit tracheobronchial suctioning to 10 to 15 seconds and should make only two passes. **(M-S)**

■ Before performing tracheobronchial suctioning, the nurse should ventilate and oxygenate the patient five to six times with a resuscitation bag and 100% oxygen. This procedure is called *bagging*. **(M-S)**

■ Signs and symptoms of pneumothorax include tachypnea, restlessness, hypotension, and tracheal deviation. **(M-S)**

■ The cardinal sign of toxic shock syndrome is rapid onset of a high fever. **(M-S)**

■ A key sign of peptic ulcer is hematemesis, which can be bright red or dark red, with the consistency of coffee grounds. **(M-S)**

Signs and symptoms of a perforated peptic ulcer include sudden, severe upper abdominal pain; vomiting; and an extremely tender, rigid (board-like) abdomen.   (M-S)

Constipation is a common adverse reaction to aluminum hydroxide.   (M-S)

For the first 24 hours after a myocardial infarction, the patient should use a bedside commode and then progress to walking to the toilet, bathing, and taking short walks.   (M-S)

After a myocardial infarction, the patient should avoid overexertion and add a new activity daily, as tolerated without dyspnea.   (M-S)

In a patient with a recent myocardial infarction, frothy, blood-tinged sputum suggests pulmonary edema.   (M-S)

In a patient who has acquired immunodeficiency syndrome, the primary purpose of drugs is to prevent secondary infections.   (M-S)

In a patient with acquired immunodeficiency syndrome, suppression of the immune system increases the risk of opportunistic infections, such as cytomegalovirus, *Pneumocystis carinii* pneumonia, and thrush.   (M-S)

A patient with acquired immunodeficiency syndrome may have rapid weight loss, a sign of *wasting syndrome.*   (M-S)

Between ages 10 and 12 months, a child begins to show emotions, such as affection, jealousy, and anger.   (PED)

Chlorpromazine (Thorazine) is used to treat neonates who are addicted to narcotics.   (MAT)

The nurse should use elbow restraints to protect an infant with eczema or a scalp vein infusion or one who is recovering from cleft lip repair or eye surgery.   (PED)

The nurse should provide a dark, quiet environment for a neonate who is experiencing narcotic withdrawal.   (MAT)

In children, the normal fasting glucose level is 60 to 100 mg/dl.   (PED)

If the body doesn't use glucose for energy, it metabolizes fat and produces ketones.   (M-S)

▓ In infants ages 6 to 12 months, separation from the mother evokes a more intense response than any other stimulus.   (PED)

▓ Because steroids mask symptoms of infection, they should be administered to children with extreme caution.   (PED)

▓ Steroids should be administered with food to a child.   (PED)

▓ Approximately 20% of patients with Guillain-Barré syndrome have residual deficits, such as mild motor weakness or diminished lower extremity reflexes.   (M-S)

▓ In children, signs and symptoms of leukemia include fatigue, anorexia, low-grade fever, and decreased white blood cell, red blood cell, and platelet counts.   (PED)

▓ In children with leukemia, the most common causes of death include hemorrhage and infection.   (PED)

▓ In a child, anemia is the first sign of lead poisoning.   (PED)

▓ A Bradford frame is commonly used to immobilize a child who has a spica cast.   (PED)

▓ In a premature neonate, signs of respiratory distress include nostril flaring, substernal retractions, and inspiratory grunting.   (MAT)

▓ Hypertension and hypokalemia are the most significant clinical manifestations of primary hyperaldosteronism.   (M-S)

▓ In a child age 3, having and frequently speaking to an imaginary friend are normal behaviors.   (PED)

▓ By age 3 to 4 months, an infant with normal motor development should be able to lift and control his head. Head lag is common in infants younger than age 3 months.   (PED)

▓ Thrush is candidiasis *(Candida albicans)* of the oral mucous membranes. It's characterized by aphthae, or small ulcers, in the mouth.   (PED)

▓ Common causes of child abuse are poor impulse control by the parents and the lack of knowledge of growth and development.   (PSY)

▓ Allopurinol (Zyloprim) is used in children with leukemia to prevent accumulation of uric acid.   (PED)

Before administering any "as needed" pain medication, the nurse should ask the patient to indicate the location of the pain.   (FND)

At age 6 months, an infant should begin to receive solid foods one at a time and 1 week apart.   (PED)

After percutaneous aspiration of the bladder, the patient's first void is usually pink; however, urine with frank blood should be reported to the physician.   (M-S)

A urine culture that grows more than 100,000 colonies of bacteria per milliliter of urine indicates infection.   (M-S)

The most appropriate toy for a toddler age 18 months is one that helps to develop motor coordination.   (PED)

When administering an injection to an infant, the nurse should ask another nurse to divert the child's attention and assist as needed.   (PED)

Respiratory distress syndrome (hyaline membrane disease) develops in premature infants because their pulmonary alveoli lack surfactant.   (MAT)

Whenever an infant is being put down to sleep, the parent or caregiver should position the infant on the back. (Remember *back to sleep.*)   (MAT)

A patient who is undergoing dialysis should take a vitamin supplement and eat foods that are high in calories, but low in protein, sodium, and potassium.   (M-S)

The nurse should communicate at eye level with a child.   (PED)

An infant who has phenylketonuria should be fed a low-phenylalanine formula and should have plasma phenylalanine levels monitored frequently.   (PED)

When caring for an infant who has had six to eight episodes of diarrhea a day for 4 days, the nurse should assess for electrolyte imbalance.   (PED)

The nurse may offer finger foods to a child age 3 who has a poor appetite.   (PED)

When in a mist tent (Croupette), a child may require soft restraints.   (PED)

- In a patient who has chronic obstructive pulmonary disease, the most effective ways to reduce thick secretions are to increase fluid intake to 2,500 ml/day and encourage ambulation. **(M-S)**

- The nurse shouldn't administer a drug to a child at bedtime unless it's specifically prescribed because it may stimulate the child. **(PED)**

- Medulloblastoma, the most common brain tumor in children, is characteristically found in the cerebellum. **(PED)**

- The nurse should teach a patient with emphysema how to perform pursed-lip breathing because this slows expiration, prevents alveolar collapse, and helps to control the respiratory rate. **(M-S)**

- Clubbing of the digits and a barrel chest may develop in a patient who has chronic obstructive pulmonary disease. **(M-S)**

- A stroke ("brain attack") disrupts the brain's blood supply and may be caused by hypertension. **(M-S)**

- In a patient who is undergoing dialysis, desired outcomes are normal weight, normal serum albumin level (3.5 to 5.5 g/dl), and adequate protein intake (1.2 to 1.5 g/kg of body weight daily). **(M-S)**

- Intermittent peritoneal dialysis involves performing three to seven treatments that total 40 hours per week. **(M-S)**

- In a patient with chronic obstructive pulmonary disease, the best way to administer oxygen is by nasal cannula. The normal flow rate is 2 to 3 L/minute. **(M-S)**

- Isoetharine (Bronkosol) can be administered with a handheld nebulizer or by intermittent positive-pressure breathing. **(M-S)**

- *Brain death* is irreversible cessation of brain function. **(M-S)**

- Continuous ambulatory peritoneal dialysis requires four exchanges per day, 7 days per week, for a total of 168 hours per week. **(M-S)**

- The classic adverse reactions to antihistamines are dry mouth, drowsiness, and blurred vision. **(M-S)**

- Because of the risk of paralytic ileus, a patient who has received a general anesthetic can't take anything by mouth until active bowel sounds are heard in all abdominal quadrants. **(M-S)**

Jehovah's Witnesses believe that they shouldn't receive blood components donated by other people.   (FND)

The level of alpha-fetoprotein, a tumor marker, is elevated in patients who have testicular germ cell cancer.   (M-S)

Clinical manifestations of orchitis caused by bacteria or mumps include high temperature, chills, and sudden pain in the involved testis.   (M-S)

The level of prostate-specific antigen is elevated in patients with benign prostatic hyperplasia or prostate cancer.   (M-S)

The level of prostatic acid phosphatase is elevated in patients with advanced stages of prostate cancer.   (M-S)

Phenylephrine (Neo-Synephrine), a mydriatic, is instilled in a patient's eye to dilate the eye.   (M-S)

To test visual acuity, the nurse should ask the patient to cover each eye separately and to read the eye chart with glasses and without, as appropriate.
                                                                        (FND)

To promote fluid drainage and relieve edema in a patient with epididymitis, the nurse should elevate the scrotum on a scrotal bridge.   (M-S)

Fluorescein staining is commonly used to assess corneal abrasions because it outlines superficial epithelial defects.   (M-S)

Presbyopia is loss of near vision as a result of the loss of elasticity of the crystalline lens.   (M-S)

When providing oral care for an unconscious patient, to minimize the risk of aspiration, the nurse should position the patient on the side.   (FND)

During assessment of distance vision, the patient should stand 20' (6.1 m) from the chart.   (FND)

Transient ischemic attacks are considered precursors to strokes.   (M-S)

A sign of acute appendicitis, McBurney's sign is tenderness at McBurney's point (about 2" [5 cm] from the right anterior superior iliac spine on a line between the spine and the umbilicus).   (M-S)

When caring for a patient with Guillain-Barré syndrome, the nurse should focus on respiratory interventions as the disease process advances.
                                                                        (M-S)

▓ The diagnosis of Alzheimer's disease is based on clinical findings of two or more cognitive deficits, progressive worsening of memory, and the results of a neuropsychological test.   (PSY)

▓ Signs and symptoms of colon cancer include rectal bleeding, change in bowel habits, intestinal obstruction, abdominal pain, weight loss, anorexia, nausea, and vomiting.   (M-S)

▓ Memory disturbance is a classic sign of Alzheimer's disease.   (PSY)

▓ To help calm a child who is frightened of a mist tent, the nurse may suggest that a parent lie with the child in the tent.   (PED)

▓ Symptoms of prostatitis include frequent urination and dysuria.   (M-S)

▓ The male sperm contributes an X or a Y chromosome; the female ovum contributes an X chromosome.   (MAT)

▓ Fertilization produces a total of 46 chromosomes, including an XY combination (male) or an XX combination (female).   (MAT)

▓ A *chancre* is a painless, ulcerative lesion that develops during the primary stage of syphilis.   (M-S)

▓ During the tertiary stage of syphilis, spirochetes invade the internal organs and cause permanent damage.   (M-S)

▓ For a geriatric patient or one who is extremely ill, the ideal room temperature is 66° to 76° F (18.8° to 24.4° C).   (FND)

▓ Normal room humidity is 30% to 60%.   (FND)

▓ Hand washing is the single best method of limiting the spread of microorganisms. Once gloves are removed after routine contact with a patient, hands should be washed for 10 to 15 seconds.   (FND)

▓ The percentage of water in a neonate's body is about 78% to 80%.
(MAT)

▓ In total parenteral nutrition, weight gain is the most reliable indicator of a positive response to therapy.   (M-S)

▓ The nurse may administer an I.V. fat emulsion through a central or peripheral catheter, but shouldn't use an in-line filter because the fat particles are too large to pass through the pores.   (M-S)

To perform catheterization, the nurse should place a woman in the dorsal recumbent position. (FND)

A positive Homans' sign may indicate thrombophlebitis. (FND)

Electrolytes in a solution are measured in milliequivalents per liter (mEq/L). A milliequivalent is the number of milligrams per 100 milliliters of a solution. (FND)

If a patient who has a prostatectomy is using a Cunningham clamp, instruct him to wash and dry his penis before applying the clamp. He should apply the clamp horizontally and remove it at least every 4 hours to empty his bladder to prevent infection. (M-S)

Thought blocking is loss of the train of thought because of a defect in mental processing. (PSY)

A Bradford frame is used for long-term immobilization of a child, such as a patient with extensive burns or meningocele. (PED)

Metabolism occurs in two phases: anabolism (the constructive phase) and catabolism (the destructive phase). (FND)

If a woman has signs of urinary tract infection during menopause, she should be instructed to drink six to eight glasses of water per day, urinate before and after intercourse, and perform Kegel exercises. (M-S)

If a menopausal patient experiences a "hot flash," she should be instructed to seek a cool, breezy location and sip a cool drink. (M-S)

The basal metabolic rate is the amount of energy needed to maintain essential body functions. It's measured when the patient is awake and resting, hasn't eaten for 14 to 18 hours, and is in a comfortable, warm environment. (FND)

The basal metabolic rate is expressed in calories consumed per hour per kilogram of body weight. (FND)

Cheilosis causes fissures at the angles of the mouth and indicates a vitamin B_2, riboflavin, or iron deficiency. (M-S)

Tetany may result from hypocalcemia caused by hypoparathyroidism. (M-S)

▓ Dietary fiber (roughage), which is derived from cellulose, supplies bulk, maintains intestinal motility, and helps to establish regular bowel habits.
(FND)

▓ Alcohol is metabolized primarily in the liver. Smaller amounts are metabolized by the kidneys and lungs.
(FND)

▓ A patient who has cervical cancer may experience vaginal bleeding for 1 to 3 months after intracavitary radiation.
(M-S)

▓ *Ascites* is the accumulation of fluid, containing large amounts of protein and electrolytes, in the abdominal cavity. It's commonly caused by cirrhosis.
(M-S)

▓ Normal pulmonary artery pressure is 10 to 25 mm Hg. Normal pulmonary artery wedge pressure is 5 to 12 mm Hg.
(M-S)

▓ After cardiac catheterization, the site is monitored for bleeding and hematoma formation, pulses distal to the site are palpated every 15 minutes for 1 hour, and the patient is maintained on bed rest with the extremity extended for 8 hours.
(M-S)

▓ *Hemophilia* is a bleeding disorder that's transmitted genetically in a sex-linked (X chromosome) recessive pattern. Although girls and women may carry the defective gene, hemophilia usually occurs only in boys and men.
(M-S)

▓ *Von Willebrand's disease* is an autosomal dominant bleeding disorder that's caused by platelet dysfunction and factor VIII deficiency.
(M-S)

▓ *Sickle cell anemia* is a congenital hemolytic anemia that's caused by defective hemoglobin S molecules. It primarily affects blacks.
(M-S)

▓ Sickle cell anemia has a homozygous inheritance pattern. Sickle cell trait has a heterozygous inheritance pattern.
(M-S)

▓ Pel-Ebstein fever is a characteristic sign of Hodgkin's disease. Fever recurs every few days or weeks and alternates with afebrile periods.
(M-S)

▓ *Petechiae* are tiny, round, purplish red spots that appear on the skin and mucous membranes as a result of intradermal or submucosal hemorrhage.
(FND)

▓ *Purpura* is a purple discoloration of the skin that's caused by blood extravasation.
(FND)

Glucose-6-phosphate dehydrogenase (G6PD) deficiency is an inherited metabolic disorder that's characterized by red blood cells that are deficient in G6PD, a critical enzyme in aerobic glycolysis.   **(M-S)**

Preferred sites for bone marrow aspiration are the posterior superior iliac crest, anterior iliac crest, and sternum.   **(M-S)**

During bone marrow harvesting, the donor receives general anesthesia and 400 to 800 ml of marrow is aspirated.   **(M-S)**

A butterfly rash across the bridge of the nose is a characteristic sign of systemic lupus erythematosus.   **(M-S)**

Rheumatoid arthritis is a chronic, destructive collagen disease characterized by symmetric inflammation of the synovium that leads to joint swelling.   **(M-S)**

A *compulsion* is an irresistible urge to perform an irrational act, such as walking in a clockwise circle before leaving a room or washing the hands repeatedly.   **(PSY)**

A patient who has a chosen method and a plan to commit suicide in the next 48 to 72 hours is at high risk for suicide.   **(PSY)**

Screening for human immunodeficiency virus antibodies begins with the enzyme-linked immunosorbent assay. Results are confirmed by the Western blot test.   **(M-S)**

The therapeutic serum level for lithium is 0.5 to 1.5 mEq/L.   **(PSY)**

Phobic disorders are treated with desensitization therapy, which gradually exposes a patient to an anxiety-producing stimulus.   **(PSY)**

Dysfunctional grieving is absent or prolonged grief.   **(PSY)**

To perform nasotracheal suctioning in an infant, the nurse positions the infant with his neck slightly hyperextended in a "sniffing" position, with his chin up and his head tilted back slightly.   **(MAT)**

To avoid hypoxia and apnea, the nurse should suction an infant quickly and gently. A longer period of suctioning may be used if the nurse administers oxygen with a handheld resuscitation bag between periods of suctioning.   **(PED)**

Organogenesis occurs during the first trimester of pregnancy, specifically, days 14 to 56 of gestation.   **(MAT)**

■ After birth, the neonate's umbilical cord is tied 1" (2.5 cm) from the abdominal wall with a cotton cord, plastic clamp, or rubber band. (MAT)

■ *Gravida* is the number of pregnancies a woman has had, regardless of outcome. (MAT)

■ *Para* is the number of pregnancies that reached viability, regardless of whether the fetus was delivered alive or stillborn. A fetus is considered viable at 20 weeks' gestation. (MAT)

■ An *ectopic pregnancy* is one that implants abnormally, outside the uterus. (MAT)

■ The first stage of labor begins with the onset of labor and ends with full cervical dilation at 10 cm. (MAT)

■ The second stage of labor begins with full cervical dilation and ends with the neonate's birth. (MAT)

■ The third stage of labor begins after the neonate's birth and ends with expulsion of the placenta. (MAT)

■ In a full-term neonate, skin creases appear over two-thirds of the neonate's feet. Preterm neonates have heel creases that cover less than two-thirds of the feet. (MAT)

■ The fourth stage of labor (postpartum stabilization) lasts up to 4 hours after the placenta is delivered. This time is needed to stabilize the mother's physical and emotional state after the stress of childbirth. (MAT)

■ At 20 weeks' gestation, the fundus is at the level of the umbilicus. (MAT)

■ At 36 weeks' gestation, the fundus is at the lower border of the rib cage. (MAT)

■ A premature neonate is one born before the end of the 37th week of gestation. (MAT)

■ The CK-MB isoenzyme level increases 4 to 8 hours after a myocardial infarction, peaks at 12 to 24 hours, and returns to normal in 3 days. (M-S)

■ During phase I of the nurse-patient relationship (beginning, or orientation, phase), the nurse obtains an initial history and the nurse and the patient agree to a contract. (PSY)

■ During phase II of the nurse-patient relationship (middle, or working, phase), the patient discusses his problems, behavioral changes occur, and self-defeating behavior is resolved or reduced. **(PSY)**

■ During phase III of the nurse-patient relationship (termination, or resolution, phase), the nurse terminates the therapeutic relationship and gives the patient positive feedback on his accomplishments. **(PSY)**

■ Pregnancy-induced hypertension is a leading cause of maternal death in the United States. **(MAT)**

■ A *habitual aborter* is a woman who has had three or more consecutive spontaneous abortions. **(MAT)**

■ *Threatened abortion* occurs when bleeding is present without cervical dilation. **(MAT)**

■ A *complete abortion* occurs when all products of conception are expelled. **(MAT)**

■ *Hydramnios* (polyhydramnios) is excessive amniotic fluid (more than 2,000 ml in the third trimester). **(MAT)**

■ Excessive intake of vitamin K may significantly antagonize the anticoagulant effects of warfarin (Coumadin). The patient should be cautioned to avoid eating an excessive amount of leafy green vegetables. **(M-S)**

■ According to the standard precautions recommended by the Centers for Disease Control and Prevention, the nurse shouldn't recap needles after use. Most needle sticks result from missed needle recapping. **(FND)**

■ According to Freud, a person between ages 12 and 20 is in the genital stage, during which he learns independence, has an increased interest in members of the opposite sex, and establishes an identity. **(PSY)**

■ According to Erikson, the identity-versus-role confusion stage occurs between ages 12 and 20. **(PSY)**

■ *Tolerance* is the need for increasing amounts of a substance to achieve an effect that formerly was achieved with lesser amounts. **(PSY)**

■ A lymph node biopsy that shows Reed-Sternberg cells provides a definitive diagnosis of Hodgkin's disease. **(M-S)**

■ The nurse should remove a child's protective mitts twice each shift to let the child exercise his fingers. **(PED)**

■ Stress, dehydration, and fatigue may reduce a breast-feeding mother's milk supply. **(MAT)**

■ *Bell's palsy* is unilateral facial weakness or paralysis caused by a disturbance of the seventh cranial (facial) nerve. **(M-S)**

■ During the transition phase of the first stage of labor, the cervix is dilated 8 to 10 cm and contractions usually occur 2 to 3 minutes apart and last for 60 seconds. **(MAT)**

■ A nonstress test is considered nonreactive (positive) if fewer than two fetal heart rate accelerations of at least 15 beats/minute occur in 20 minutes. **(MAT)**

■ A nonstress test is considered reactive (negative) if two or more fetal heart rate accelerations of 15 beats/minute above baseline occur in 20 minutes. **(MAT)**

■ A nonstress test is usually performed to assess fetal well-being in a pregnant patient with a prolonged pregnancy (42 weeks or more), diabetes, a history of poor pregnancy outcomes, or pregnancy-induced hypertension. **(MAT)**

■ The nurse administers a drug by I.V. push by using a needle and syringe to deliver the dose directly into a vein, I.V. tubing, or a catheter. **(FND)**

■ When feeding an infant who has a tracheostomy tube, the nurse should cover the opening of the tracheostomy tube (stoma) with moistened gauze. A bib may be used for a child older than age 1. **(PED)**

■ When changing the ties on a tracheostomy tube, the nurse should leave the old ties in place until the new ones are applied. **(FND)**

■ A nurse should have assistance when changing the ties on a tracheostomy tube. **(FND)**

■ To change a diaper, a nurse shouldn't lift an infant by the legs. The nurse should roll the infant to the side, put the diaper in place, and then roll the infant onto the diaper. **(PED)**

■ A spica cast dries completely in 24 to 72 hours. **(PED)**

During an initial tuberculin skin test, lack of a wheal after injection of tuberculin purified protein derivative indicates that the test dose was injected too deeply. The nurse should inject another dose at least 2" (5 cm) from the initial site.   (M-S)

A tuberculin skin test should be read 48 to 72 hours after administration.   (M-S)

In reading a tuberculin skin test, erythema without induration is usuallyn't significant.   (M-S)

Death caused by botulism usually results from delayed diagnosis and respiratory complications.   (M-S)

In a patient who has rabies, saliva contains the virus and is a hazard for nurses who provide care.   (M-S)

A pregnant woman should drink at least eight 8-oz glasses (about 2,000 ml) of water daily.   (MAT)

A filter is always used for blood transfusions.   (FND)

A febrile nonhemolytic reaction is the most common transfusion reaction.   (M-S)

A four-point (quad) cane is indicated when a patient needs more stability than a regular cane can provide.   (FND)

A good way to begin a patient interview is to ask, "What made you seek medical help?"   (FND)

When caring for any patient, the nurse should follow standard precautions for handling blood and body fluids.   (FND)

Potassium (K^+) is the most abundant cation in intracellular fluid.
                                                                        (FND)

Hypokalemia (abnormally low concentration of potassium in the blood) may cause muscle weakness or paralysis, electrocardiographic abnormalities, and GI disturbances.   (M-S)

In the four-point, or alternating, gait, the patient first moves the right crutch followed by the left foot and then the left crutch followed by the right foot.   (FND)

In the three-point gait, the patient moves two crutches and the affected leg simultaneously and then moves the unaffected leg. (FND)

In the two-point gait, the patient moves the right leg and the left crutch simultaneously and then moves the left leg and the right crutch simultaneously. (FND)

The vitamin B complex, the water-soluble vitamins that are essential for metabolism, include thiamine (B_1), riboflavin (B_2), niacin (B_3), pyridoxine (B_6), and cyanocobalamin (B_{12}). (FND)

When being weighed, an adult patient should be lightly dressed and shoeless. (FND)

Beriberi, a serious vitamin B_1 (thiamine) deficiency, affects alcoholics who have poor dietary habits. It's epidemic in Asian countries where people subsist on unenriched rice. It's characterized by the phrase "I can't," indicating that the patient is too ill to do anything. (M-S)

Before taking an adult's temperature orally, the nurse should ensure that the patient hasn't smoked or consumed hot or cold substances in the previous 15 minutes. (FND)

The nurse shouldn't take an adult's temperature rectally if the patient has a cardiac disorder, anal lesions, or bleeding hemorrhoids or has recently undergone rectal surgery. (FND)

Excessive sedation may cause respiratory depression. (M-S)

In a patient who has a cardiac disorder, measuring temperature rectally may stimulate a vagal response and lead to vasodilation and decreased cardiac output. (FND)

When recording pulse amplitude and rhythm, the nurse should use these descriptive measures: +3, bounding pulse (readily palpable and forceful); +2, normal pulse (easily palpable); +1, thready or weak pulse (difficult to detect); and 0, absent pulse (not detectable). (FND)

A preoperative method used to teach a child about postoperative events is to describe these events using a life-size doll that has an incision, a dressing, a cast, or an I.V. line, as appropriate. (PED)

The intraoperative period begins when a patient is transferred to the operating room bed and ends when the patient is admitted to the postanesthesia care unit. (FND)

On the morning of surgery, the nurse should ensure that the informed consent form has been signed; that the patient hasn't taken anything by mouth since midnight, has taken a shower with antimicrobial soap, has had mouth care (without swallowing the water), has removed common jewelry, and has received preoperative medication as prescribed; and that vital signs have been taken and recorded. Artificial limbs and other prostheses are usually removed.   (FND)

The primary postoperative concern is maintenance of a patent airway.
                                                                    (M-S)

If cyanosis occurs circumorally, sublingually, or in the nail bed, the oxygen saturation level (SaO_2) is less than 80%.   (M-S)

A rapid pulse rate in a postoperative patient may indicate pain, bleeding, dehydration, or shock.   (M-S)

Increased pulse rate and blood pressure may indicate that a patient is experiencing "silent pain" (pain that can't be expressed verbally, such as when a patient is recovering from anesthesia).   (M-S)

Lidocaine (Xylocaine) exerts antiarrhythmic action by suppressing automaticity in the Purkinje fibers and elevating the electrical stimulation threshold in the ventricles.   (M-S)

Cullen's sign (a bluish discoloration around the umbilicus) is seen in patients who have a perforated pancreas.   (M-S)

Comfort measures, such as positioning the patient, rubbing the patient's back, and providing a restful environment, may decrease the patient's need for analgesics or may enhance their effectiveness.   (FND)

During the postoperative period, the patient should cough and breathe deeply every 2 hours unless otherwise contraindicated (for example, after craniotomy, cataract surgery, or throat surgery).   (M-S)

Before surgery, a patient's respiratory volume may be measured by incentive spirometry. This measurement becomes the patient's postoperative goal for respiratory volume.   (M-S)

The postoperative patient should use incentive spirometry 10 to 12 times per hour and breathe deeply.   (M-S)

Before ambulating, a postoperative patient should dangle his legs over the side of the bed and perform deep-breathing exercises.   (M-S)

During the patient's first postoperative ambulation, the nurse should monitor the patient closely and assist him as needed while he walks a few feet from the bed to a steady chair. (M-S)

Hypovolemia occurs when 15% to 25% of the body's total blood volume is lost. (M-S)

Signs and symptoms of hypovolemia include rapid, weak pulse; low blood pressure; cool, clammy skin; shallow respirations; oliguria or anuria; and lethargy. (M-S)

Acute pericarditis causes sudden severe, constant pain over the anterior chest. The pain is aggravated by inspiration. (M-S)

Signs and symptoms of septicemia include fever, chills, rash, abdominal distention, prostration, pain, headache, nausea, and diarrhea. (M-S)

Rocky Mountain spotted fever causes a persistent high fever, nonpitting edema, and rash. (M-S)

Patients who have undergone coronary artery bypass graft should sleep 6 to 10 hours per day, take their temperature twice daily, and avoid lifting more than 10 lb (4.5 kg) for at least 6 weeks. (M-S)

Claudication pain (pain on ambulation) is caused by arterial insufficiency as a result of atheromatous plaque that obstructs arterial blood flow to the extremities. (M-S)

When both breasts are used for breast-feeding, the infant usually doesn't empty the second breast. Therefore, the second breast should be used first at the next feeding. (MAT)

Pacemakers can be powered by lithium batteries for up to 10 years. (M-S)

The patient shouldn't void for 1 hour before percutaneous suprapubic bladder aspiration to ensure that sufficient urine remains in the bladder to make the procedure successful. (M-S)

Left-sided heart failure causes pulmonary congestion, pink-tinged sputum, and dyspnea. (Remember *L* for *left* and *lung*.) (M-S)

When placing a rubber band tourniquet on an infant's head before starting a scalp vein infusion, the nurse should place a second rubber band crosswise under the band to facilitate lifting and cutting the tourniquet when it's removed. **(PED)**

A low-birth-weight neonate weighs 2,500 g (5 lb 8 oz) or less at birth. **(MAT)**

A very-low-birth-weight neonate weighs 1,500 g (3 lb 5 oz) or less at birth. **(MAT)**

When lifting an infant, the nurse should maintain two points of contact with the infant's body at all times. **(PED)**

When teaching parents to provide umbilical cord care, the nurse should teach them to clean the umbilical area with a cotton ball saturated with alcohol after every diaper change to prevent infection and promote drying. **(MAT)**

Parents of young children should set the thermostat on their water heater no higher than 130° F (54° C). **(PED)**

Suicide is the third leading cause of death among white teenagers. **(PSY)**

Most teenagers who kill themselves made a previous suicide attempt and left telltale signs of their plans. **(PSY)**

The nurse should teach a teenage girl that the most effective birth control method is abstinence and that the second most effective method is oral contraceptive use. **(PED)**

Teenage mothers are more likely to have low-birth-weight neonates because they seek prenatal care late in pregnancy (as a result of denial) and are more likely than older mothers to have nutritional deficiencies. **(MAT)**

The current recommended blood cholesterol level is less than 200 mg/dl. **(M-S)**

▓ When caring for a patient who is having a seizure, the nurse should follow these guidelines: (1) Avoid restraining the patient, but help a standing patient to a lying position. (2) Loosen restrictive clothing. (3) Place a pillow or another soft object under the patient's head. (4) Clear the area of hard objects. (5) Don't force anything into the patient's mouth, but maintain a patent airway. (6) Reassure and reorient the patient after the seizure subsides. (M-S)

▓ Gingival hyperplasia, or overgrowth of gum tissue, is an adverse reaction to phenytoin (Dilantin). (M-S)

▓ A drug has three names: generic name, which is used in official publications; trade, or brand, name (such as Tylenol), which is selected by the drug company; and chemical name, which describes the drug's chemical composition. (FND)

▓ To avoid staining the teeth, the patient should take a liquid iron preparation through a straw. (FND)

▓ The nurse should use the Z-track method to administer an I.M. injection of iron dextran (Imferon). (FND)

▓ An organism may enter the body through the nose, mouth, rectum, urinary or reproductive tract, or skin. (FND)

▓ With aging, most marrow in long bones becomes yellow, but it retains the capacity to convert back to red. (M-S)

▓ Clinical manifestations of lymphedema include accumulation of fluid in the legs. (M-S)

▓ *Afterload* is ventricular wall tension during systolic ejection. It's increased in patients who have septal hypertrophy, increased blood viscosity, and conditions that cause blockage of aortic or pulmonary outflow. (M-S)

▓ Red blood cells can be stored frozen for up to 2 years; however, they must be used within 24 hours of thawing. (M-S)

▓ *Linea nigra*, a dark line that extends from the umbilicus to the mons pubis, commonly appears during pregnancy and disappears after pregnancy. (MAT)

▓ Implantation in the uterus occurs 6 to 10 days after ovum fertilization. (MAT)

In Erikson's stage of generativity versus despair, generativity (investment of the self in the interest of the larger community) is expressed through procreation, work, community service, and creative endeavors. **(PSY)**

Most infants double their birth weight by age 5 to 6 months and triple it by age 1 year. **(PED)**

For the first 24 hours after amputation, the nurse should elevate the stump to prevent edema. **(M-S)**

After hysterectomy, a woman should avoid sexual intercourse for 3 weeks if a vaginal approach was used and 6 weeks if the abdominal approach was used. **(M-S)**

In descending order, the levels of consciousness are alertness, lethargy, stupor, light coma, and deep coma. **(FND)**

Parkinson's disease characteristically causes progressive muscle rigidity, akinesia, and involuntary tremor. **(M-S)**

Tonic-clonic seizures are characterized by a loss of consciousness and alternating periods of muscle contraction and relaxation. **(M-S)**

Status epilepticus, a life-threatening emergency, is a series of rapidly repeating seizures that occur without intervening periods of consciousness. **(M-S)**

The ideal donor for kidney transplantation is an identical twin. If an identical twin isn't available, a biological sibling is the next best choice. **(M-S)**

Breast cancer is the leading cancer among women; however, lung cancer accounts for more deaths. **(M-S)**

The stages of cervical cancer are as follows: stage 0, carcinoma in situ; stage I, cancer confined to the cervix; stage II, cancer extending beyond the cervix, but not to the pelvic wall; stage III, cancer extending to the pelvic wall; and stage IV, cancer extending beyond the pelvis or within the bladder or rectum. **(M-S)**

One method used to estimate blood loss after a hysterectomy is counting perineal pads. Saturating more than one pad in 1 hour or eight pads in 24 hours is considered hemorrhaging. **(M-S)**

Transurethral resection of the prostate is the most common procedure for treating benign prostatic hyperplasia. **(M-S)**

In a chest drainage system, the water in the water-seal chamber normally rises when a patient breathes in and falls when he breathes out. **(M-S)**

Placenta previa is abnormally low implantation of the placenta so that it encroaches on or covers the cervical os. **(MAT)**

Spinal fusion provides spinal stability through a bone graft, usually from the iliac crest, that fuses two or more vertebrae. **(M-S)**

To turn a patient by logrolling, the nurse folds the patient's arms across the chest; extends the patient's legs and inserts a pillow between them, if needed; places a draw sheet under the patient; and turns the patient by slowly and gently pulling on the draw sheet. **(FND)**

In complete (total) placenta previa, the placenta completely covers the cervical os. **(MAT)**

In partial (incomplete or marginal) placenta previa, the placenta covers only a portion of the cervical os. **(MAT)**

A patient who receives any type of transplant must take an immunosuppressant drug for the rest of his life. **(M-S)**

Abruptio placentae is premature separation of a normally implanted placenta. It may be partial or complete, and usually causes abdominal pain, vaginal bleeding, and a boardlike abdomen. **(MAT)**

Cutis marmorata is mottling or purple discoloration of the skin. It's a transient vasomotor response that occurs primarily in the arms and legs of infants who are exposed to cold. **(MAT)**

The classic triad of symptoms of preeclampsia are hypertension, edema, and proteinuria. Additional symptoms of severe preeclampsia include hyperreflexia, cerebral and vision disturbances, and epigastric pain. **(MAT)**

Incentive spirometry should be used 5 to 10 times an hour while the patient is awake. **(M-S)**

In a male patient who has reached puberty, the major complication of mumps is sterility caused by orchitis. **(PED)**

In women, pelvic inflammatory disease is a common complication of gonorrhea. (M-S)

Hirschsprung's disease (congenital megacolon) is the congenital absence of parasympathetic ganglia in the distal portion of the colon and rectum, which results in a lack of peristalsis. (PED)

Ortolani's sign (an audible click or palpable jerk that occurs with thigh abduction) confirms congenital hip dislocation in a neonate. (MAT)

Scoliosis is lateral S-shaped curvature of the spine. (M-S)

According to Freud, conflicts that arise in the phallic stage (Oedipus or Electra complex) are resolved when the child identifies with the parent of the same sex. (PED)

Signs and symptoms of the secondary stage of syphilis include a rash on the palms and soles, erosion of the oral mucosa, alopecia, and enlarged lymph nodes. (M-S)

Alcoholics Anonymous recommends a 12-step program to achieve sobriety. (PSY)

In a patient who is receiving total parenteral nutrition, the nurse should monitor glucose and electrolyte levels. (M-S)

Signs and symptoms of anorexia nervosa include amenorrhea, excessive weight loss, lanugo (fine body hair), abdominal distention, and electrolyte disturbances. (PSY)

Unless contraindicated, on admission to the postanesthesia care unit, a patient should be turned on his side and his vital signs should be taken. (M-S)

Edema is treated by limiting fluid intake and eliminating excess fluid. (M-S)

A patient who has had spinal anesthesia should remain flat for 12 to 24 hours. Vital signs and neuromuscular function should be monitored. (M-S)

A serum lithium level that exceeds 2.0 mEq/L is considered toxic. (PSY)

A patient who has maple syrup urine disease should avoid food containing the amino acids leucine, isoleucine, and lysine. (M-S)

■ A severe complication of a femur fracture is excessive blood loss that results in shock. **(M-S)**

■ To prepare a patient for peritoneal dialysis, the nurse should ask the patient to void, measure his vital signs, place him in a supine position, and using aseptic technique, insert a catheter through the abdominal wall and into the peritoneal space. **(M-S)**

■ If more than 3 L of dialysate solution return during peritoneal dialysis, the nurse should notify the physician. **(M-S)**

■ *Hemodialysis* is the removal of certain elements from the blood by passing heparinized blood through a semipermeable membrane to the dialysate bath, which contains all of the important electrolytes in their ideal concentrations. **(M-S)**

■ The first immunization for a neonate is the hepatitis B vaccine, which is administered in the nursery shortly after birth. **(MAT)**

■ Gangrene usually affects the digits first, and begins with skin color changes that progress from gray-blue to dark brown or black. **(M-S)**

■ Kidney function is assessed by evaluating blood urea nitrogen (normal range is 8 to 20 mg/dl) and serum creatinine (normal range is 0.6 to 1.3 mg/dl) levels. **(M-S)**

■ The diaphragm of the stethoscope is used to hear high-pitched sounds, such as breath sounds. **(FND)**

■ A slight difference in blood pressure (5 to 10 mm Hg) between the right and the left arms is normal. **(FND)**

■ A weight-bearing transfer is appropriate only for a patient who has at least one leg that's strong enough to bear weight, such as a patient with hemiplegia or a single-leg amputation. **(M-S)**

■ The nurse should place the blood pressure cuff 1″ (2.5 cm) above the antecubital fossa. **(FND)**

■ When instilling ophthalmic ointments, the nurse should waste the first bead of ointment and then apply the ointment from the inner canthus to the outer canthus. **(FND)**

■ The nurse should use a leg cuff to measure blood pressure in an obese patient. **(FND)**

- If a blood pressure cuff is applied too loosely, the reading will be falsely elevated. **(FND)**

- *Ptosis* is drooping of the eyelid. **(FND)**

- Overflow incontinence (voiding of 30 to 60 ml of urine every 15 to 30 minutes) is a sign of bladder distention. **(M-S)**

- The first sign of a pressure ulcer is reddened skin that blanches when pressure is applied. **(M-S)**

- A tilt table is useful for a patient with a spinal cord injury, orthostatic hypotension, or brain damage because it can move the patient gradually from a horizontal to a vertical (upright) position. **(FND)**

- To perform venipuncture with the least injury to the vessel, the nurse should turn the bevel upward when the vessel's lumen is larger than the needle and turn it downward when the lumen is only slightly larger than the needle. **(FND)**

- To move a patient to the edge of the bed for transfer, the nurse should follow these steps: Move the patient's head and shoulders toward the edge of the bed. Move the patient's feet and legs to the edge of the bed (crescent position). Place both arms well under the patient's hips, and straighten the back while moving the patient toward the edge of the bed. **(FND)**

- Late signs and symptoms of sickle cell anemia include tachycardia, cardiomegaly, systolic and diastolic murmurs, chronic fatigue, hepatomegaly, and splenomegaly. **(M-S)**

- During early childhood, signs and symptoms of sickle cell anemia include jaundice, pallor, joint swelling, bone pain, chest pain, ischemic leg ulcers, and increased susceptibility to infection. **(PED)**

- When being measured for crutches, a patient should wear shoes. **(FND)**

- If a patient misses a menstrual period while taking an oral contraceptive exactly as prescribed, she should continue taking the contraceptive.
  (MAT)

- If a patient misses two consecutive menstrual periods while taking an oral contraceptive, she should discontinue the contraceptive and take a pregnancy test. **(MAT)**

If a patient who is taking an oral contraceptive misses a dose, she should take the pill as soon as she remembers or take two at the next scheduled interval and continue with the normal schedule.   (MAT)

If a patient who is taking an oral contraceptive misses two consecutive doses, she should double the dose for 2 days and then resume her normal schedule. She also should use an additional birth control method for 1 week.   (MAT)

A mechanical ventilator, which can maintain ventilation automatically for an extended period, is indicated when a patient can't maintain a safe Pao_2 or $Paco_2$ level.   (M-S)

Two types of mechanical ventilators exist: negative-pressure ventilators, which apply negative pressure around the chest wall, and positive-pressure ventilators, which deliver air under pressure to the patient.   (M-S)

Angina pectoris is characterized by substernal pain that lasts for 2 to 3 minutes. The pain, which is caused by myocardial ischemia, may radiate to the neck, shoulders, or jaw; is described as viselike, or constricting; and may be accompanied by severe apprehension or a feeling of impending doom.   (M-S)

The diagnosis of an acute myocardial infarction is based on the patient's signs and symptoms, electrocardiogram tracings, troponin level, and cardiac enzyme studies.   (M-S)

The goal of treatment for a patient with angina pectoris is to reduce the heart's workload, thereby reducing the myocardial demand for oxygen and preventing myocardial infarction.   (M-S)

Nitroglycerin decreases the amount of blood that returns to the heart by increasing the capacity of the venous bed.   (M-S)

The patient should take no more than three nitroglycerin tablets in a 15-minute period.   (M-S)

Hemodialysis is usually performed 24 hours before kidney transplantation.   (M-S)

Signs and symptoms of acute kidney transplant rejection are progressive enlargement and tenderness at the transplant site, increased blood pressure, decreased urine output, elevated serum creatinine level, and fever.   (M-S)

In an infant, one of the first signs of dehydration is sunken fontanels.
(PED)

After a radical mastectomy, the patient's arm should be elevated (with the hand above the elbow) on a pillow to enhance circulation and prevent edema. **(M-S)**

Postoperative mastectomy care includes teaching the patient arm exercises to facilitate lymph drainage and prevent shortening of the muscle and contracture of the shoulder joint (frozen shoulder). **(M-S)**

Eclampsia is the occurrence of seizures that aren't caused by a cerebral disorder in a patient who has pregnancy-induced hypertension. **(MAT)**

After radical mastectomy, the patient should help prevent infection by making sure that no blood pressure readings, injections, or venipunctures are performed on the affected arm. **(M-S)**

In placenta previa, bleeding is painless and seldom fatal on the first occasion, but it becomes heavier with each subsequent episode. **(MAT)**

For a patient who has undergone mastectomy and is susceptible to lymphedema, a program of hand exercises can begin shortly after surgery, if prescribed. The program consists of opening and closing the hand tightly six to eight times per hour and performing such tasks as washing the face and combing the hair. **(M-S)**

Treatment for abruptio placentae is usually immediate cesarean delivery.
(MAT)

The nurse shouldn't hand-carry a hospitalized infant or child. The patient should be transported in a stroller, wheelchair, or bed. **(PED)**

The nurse should attach a restraint to the part of the bed frame that moves with the head, not to the mattress or side rails. **(FND)**

Drugs used to treat withdrawal symptoms in neonates include phenobarbital (Luminal), camphorated opium tincture (paregoric), and diazepam (Valium). **(MAT)**

Signs and symptoms of theophylline toxicity include vomiting, restlessness, and an apical pulse rate of more than 200 beats/minute. **(M-S)**

The mist in a mist tent should never become so dense that it obscures clear visualization of the patient's respiratory pattern. **(FND)**

■ The nurse should teach the parent of a child who has croup not to administer cough medication because it may worsen the child's respiratory distress by inhibiting the body's natural response to clear the throat by coughing. **(PED)**

■ Infants with Down syndrome typically have marked hypotonia, floppiness, slanted eyes, excess skin on the back of the neck, flattened bridge of the nose, flat facial features, spadelike hands, short and broad feet, small male genitalia, absence of Moro's reflex, and a simian crease on the hands. **(MAT)**

■ The nurse shouldn't induce vomiting in a person who has ingested poison and is having seizures or is semiconscious or comatose. **(M-S)**

■ Public Law 94-247 (Child Abuse and Neglect Act of 1973) requires reporting of suspected cases of child abuse to child protection services. **(PSY)**

■ The nurse should suspect sexual abuse in a young child who has blood in the feces or urine, penile or vaginal discharge, genital trauma that isn't readily explained, or a sexually transmitted disease. **(PSY)**

■ Central venous pressure (CVP), which is the pressure in the right atrium and the great veins of the thorax, is normally 2 to 8 mm Hg (or 5 to 12 cm H_2O). CVP is used to assess right-sided cardiac function. **(M-S)**

■ CVP is monitored to assess the need for fluid replacement in seriously ill patients, to estimate blood volume deficits, and to evaluate circulatory pressure in the right atrium. **(M-S)**

■ To administer heparin subcutaneously, the nurse should follow these steps: Clean, but don't rub, the site with alcohol. Stretch the skin taut or pick up a well-defined skin fold. Hold the shaft of the needle in a dart position. Insert the needle into the skin at a right (90-degree) angle. Firmly depress the plunger, but don't aspirate. Leave the needle in place for 10 seconds. Withdraw the needle gently at the angle of insertion. Apply pressure to the injection site with an alcohol pad. **(FND)**

■ To prevent deep vein thrombosis after surgery, the nurse should administer 5,000 units of heparin subcutaneously every 8 to 12 hours, as prescribed. **(M-S)**

■ Oral anticoagulants, such as warfarin (Coumadin) and dicumarol, disrupt natural blood clotting mechanisms, prevent thrombus formation, and limit the extension of a formed thrombus. **(M-S)**

■ Anticoagulants can't dissolve a formed thrombus. **(M-S)**

■ Anticoagulant therapy is contraindicated in a patient who has liver or kidney disease or GI ulcers or who isn't likely to return for follow-up visits. **(M-S)**

■ The nurse can assess a patient for thrombophlebitis by measuring the affected and unaffected legs and comparing their sizes. The nurse should mark the measurement locations with a pen so that the legs can be measured at the same place each day. **(M-S)**

■ Drainage of more than 3,000 ml of fluid daily from a nasogastric tube may suggest intestinal obstruction. Yellow drainage that has a foul odor may indicate small-bowel obstruction. **(M-S)**

■ For a sigmoidoscopy, the nurse should place the patient in the knee-chest position or Sims' position, depending on the physician's preference. **(FND)**

■ Preparation for sigmoidoscopy includes administering an enema 1 hour before the examination, warming the scope in warm water or a sterilizer (if using a metal sigmoidoscope), and draping the patient to expose the perineum. **(M-S)**

■ Treatment for a patient with bleeding esophageal varices includes administering vasopressin (Pitressin), giving an ice water lavage, aspirating blood from the stomach, using esophageal balloon tamponade, providing parenteral nutrition, and administering blood transfusions, as needed. **(M-S)**

■ A trauma victim shouldn't be moved until a patent airway is established and the cervical spine is immobilized. **(M-S)**

■ After a mastectomy, lymphedema may cause a feeling of heaviness in the affected arm. **(M-S)**

■ A school-age child who is faced with dying should be told the truth. The diagnosis should be explained to the child, and he should be allowed to die in comfort, surrounded by his family. **(PED)**

- A preschool-age child who has a fatal disease isn't likely to ask if he's going to die, but may express anxiety about death through play therapy or other activities. Most developmental theorists recommend helping the child by answering the child's questions honestly and reassuring him that he won't be alone. **(PED)**

- It's appropriate for the parents and family of a dying child to tell the child that they will miss him and that they are sad because they will be separated. **(PED)**

- An adolescent who has a terminal illness should be told the truth about his prognosis. Resentment and denial ("Is it possible that I will live?") are common responses. **(PED)**

- A dying patient shouldn't be told exactly how long he's expected to live, but should be told something more general such as "Some people live 3 to 6 months, but others live longer." **(M-S)**

- After a child dies, the nurse should give the family members time with the body, compliment them (as appropriate) on the excellent care that they provided, and give them the name of a person to contact if they have questions. **(PED)**

- *Amniocentesis* is needle aspiration of amniotic fluid. It's usually performed at 15 to 17 weeks' gestation to detect fetal abnormalities. **(MAT)**

- For a child older than age 1 who has ingested a noncorrosive poison, treatment includes administration of 15 ml of syrup of ipecac mixed in warm water. If the first dose is ineffective, a second dose may be ordered by the physician. Tincture of ipecac shouldn't be used because it's stronger than syrup of ipecac and is itself a poison. **(PED)**

- After eye surgery, a patient should avoid using makeup until otherwise instructed. **(M-S)**

- After a corneal transplant, the patient should wear an eye shield when engaging in activities such as playing with children or pets. **(M-S)**

- After a corneal transplant, the patient shouldn't lie on the affected site, bend at the waist, or have sexual intercourse for 1 week. The patient must avoid getting soapsuds in the eye. **(M-S)**

- An alcoholic uses alcohol to cope with the stresses of life. **(PSY)**

■ Theophylline, steroids, and terbutaline are commonly used to treat children with asthma. (PED)

■ Treatment of a child with celiac disease includes following a lifelong gluten-free diet. Gluten is found in wheat, oats, and barley. (PED)

■ The *ectoderm* is the outermost layer of the three primary germ layers of the embryo. (MAT)

■ The human personality operates on three levels: conscious, preconscious, and unconscious. (PSY)

■ Asking a patient an open-ended question is one of the best ways to elicit or clarify information. (PSY)

■ The failure rate of a contraceptive is determined by the experience of 100 women for 1 year. It's expressed as pregnancies per 100 woman-years. (MAT)

■ The narrowest diameter of the pelvic inlet is the anteroposterior (diagonal conjugate). (MAT)

■ The *chorion* is the outermost extraembryonic membrane that gives rise to the placenta. (MAT)

■ The corpus luteum secretes large quantities of progesterone. (MAT)

■ From the 8th week of gestation through delivery, the developing cells are known as a *fetus*. (MAT)

■ The diagnosis of autism is often made when a child is between ages 2 and 3. (PSY)

■ In an incomplete abortion, the fetus is expelled, but parts of the placenta and membrane remain in the uterus. (MAT)

■ The circumference of a neonate's head is normally 2 to 3 cm greater than the circumference of the chest. (MAT)

■ After administering magnesium sulfate to a pregnant patient for hypertension or preterm labor, the nurse should monitor the respiratory rate and deep tendon reflexes. (MAT)

■ During the first hour after birth (the period of reactivity), the neonate is alert and awake. (MAT)

When a pregnant patient has undiagnosed vaginal bleeding, vaginal examination should be avoided until ultrasonography rules out placenta previa.   (MAT)

After delivery, the first nursing action is to establish the neonate's airway.   (MAT)

Nursing interventions for a patient with placenta previa include positioning the patient on her left side for maximum fetal perfusion, monitoring fetal heart tones, and administering I.V. fluids and oxygen, as ordered.   (MAT)

When taking a child's temperature rectally, the nurse should insert the thermometer only 1½" (3.8 cm).   (PED)

The specific gravity of a neonate's urine is 1.003 to 1.030. A lower specific gravity suggests overhydration; a higher one suggests dehydration.   (MAT)

During the oral stage of development (from age 1 to 18 months), the infant receives satisfaction, relieves tension, and derives pleasure from sucking and chewing.   (PED)

Defense mechanisms protect the personality by reducing stress and anxiety.   (PSY)

A *Milwaukee brace* is used for patients who have structural scoliosis. The brace helps to halt the progression of spinal curvature by providing longitudinal traction and lateral pressure. It should be worn 23 hours a day.   (M-S)

Suppression is voluntary exclusion of stress-producing thoughts from the consciousness.   (PSY)

For the first 6 months of life, most infants are weighed and measured monthly.   (PED)

The neonatal period extends from birth to day 28. It's also called the first 4 weeks or first month of life.   (MAT)

The infancy period lasts from birth to age 1.   (PED)

The toddler stage encompasses ages 1 to 3.   (PED)

Children who have chronic protein-calorie malnutrition are small for their age, physically inactive, mentally sluggish, and susceptible to infection.   (PED)

Short-term measures used to treat stomal retraction include stool softeners, irrigation, and stomal dilatation.   (M-S)

A woman who is breast-feeding should rub a mild emollient cream or a few drops of breast milk (or colostrum) on the nipples after each feeding. She should let the breasts air-dry to prevent them from cracking.
                                                                        (MAT)

Breast-feeding mothers should increase their fluid intake to $2\frac{1}{2}$ to 3 qt (2,500 to 3,000 ml) daily.   (MAT)

In *psychodrama*, life situations are approximated in a structured environment, allowing the participant to recreate and enact scenes to gain insight and to practice new skills.   (PSY)

Psychodrama is a therapeutic technique that's used with groups to help participants gain new perception and self-awareness by acting out their own or assigned problems.   (PSY)

Maslow's hierarchy of needs must be met in the following order: physiologic (oxygen, food, water, sex, rest, and comfort), safety and security, love and belonging, self-esteem and recognition, and self-actualization.
                                                                        (FND)

A patient who is taking disulfiram (Antabuse) must avoid ingesting products that contain alcohol, such as cough syrup, fruitcake, and sauces and soups made with cooking wine.   (PSY)

A patient who is admitted to a psychiatric hospital involuntarily loses the right to sign out against medical advice.   (PSY)

"People who live in glass houses shouldn't throw stones" and "A rolling stone gathers no moss" are examples of proverbs used during a psychiatric interview to determine a patient's ability to think abstractly. (Schizophrenic patients think in concrete terms and might interpret the glass house proverb as "If you throw a stone in a glass house, the house will break.")   (PSY)

Signs of lithium toxicity include diarrhea, tremors, nausea, muscle weakness, ataxia, and confusion.   (PSY)

▦ A labile affect is characterized by rapid shifts of emotions and mood.
(PSY)

▦ *Amnesia* is loss of memory from an organic or inorganic cause. (PSY)

▦ A person who has borderline personality disorder is demanding and judg-
mental in interpersonal relationships and will attempt to split staff by
pointing to discrepancies in the treatment plan. (PSY)

▦ Disulfiram (Antabuse) shouldn't be taken concurrently with metronidazole (Flagyl) because they may interact and cause a psychotic reaction. (PSY)

▦ In patients younger than age 3, developmental dysplasia of the hip is the
most common disorder of the hip. (PED)

▦ A patient who has a colostomy should be advised to eat a low-residue
diet for 4 to 6 weeks and then to add one food at a time to evaluate its
effect. (M-S)

▦ To relieve postoperative hiccups, the patient should breathe into a paper
bag. (M-S)

▦ If a patient with an ileostomy has a blocked lumen as a result of undi-
gested high-fiber food, the patient should be placed in the knee-chest
position and the area below the stoma should be massaged. (M-S)

▦ After feeding an infant with a cleft lip or palate, the nurse should rinse
the infant's mouth with sterile water. (MAT)

▦ An infant with a cleft palate is at increased risk for otitis media. (PED)

▦ When examining an infant's ear with an otoscope, the nurse should pull
the earlobe down and back. (PED)

▦ In an infant who has had corrective surgery for a cleft lip or palate, the
nurse should place oral medication in the side of the mouth. (PED)

▦ The nurse should position a child with meningococcal meningitis on the
side if opisthotonos (back arching) occurs. (PED)

▦ Between ages 2 and 3, a child engages in parallel play and begins to interact with others. (PED)

■ For a child who has ascites as a result of chronic liver disease, the nurse should use the semi-Fowler position to promote respiratory functioning.

(PED)

■ An autistic child is difficult to understand because of withdrawal, unresponsiveness, and severely impaired speech. (PED)

■ In a toddler, the first signs of respiratory distress are increased respiratory and pulse rates. (PED)

■ Toilet training is usually unsuccessful before ages 15 to 18 months because sphincter control develops at this age. (PED)

■ The nurse instills erythromycin in a neonate's eyes primarily to prevent blindness caused by gonorrhea or chlamydia. (MAT)

■ Gonorrhea is asymptomatic and progresses without detection in most teenage girls; as a result, the fallopian tubes can be damaged. (PED)

■ During the initial interview and treatment of a patient with syphilis, the patient's sexual contacts should be identified. (M-S)

■ The nurse shouldn't administer morphine to a patient whose respiratory rate is less than 12 breaths/minute. (M-S)

■ To prevent drying of the mucous membranes, oxygen should be administered with hydration. (M-S)

■ Flavoxate (Urispas) is classified as a urinary tract spasmolytic. (M-S)

■ Hypotension is a sign of cardiogenic shock in a patient with a myocardial infarction. (M-S)

■ The predominant signs of mechanical ileus are cramping pain, vomiting, distention, and inability to pass feces or flatus. (M-S)

■ For a patient with a myocardial infarction, the nurse should monitor fluid intake and output meticulously. Too little intake causes dehydration, and too much may cause pulmonary edema. (M-S)

■ Nitroglycerin relaxes smooth muscle, causing vasodilation and relieving the chest pain associated with myocardial infarction and angina. (M-S)

■ The diagnosis of an acute myocardial infarction is based on the patient's signs and symptoms, electrocardiogram tracings, and serum enzyme studies. (M-S)

■ Arrhythmias are the predominant problem during the first 48 hours after a myocardial infarction. (M-S)

■ Clinical manifestations of malabsorption include weight loss, muscle wasting, bloating, and steatorrhea. (M-S)

■ When caring for a patient who has a nasogastric tube, the nurse should apply a water-soluble lubricant to the nostril to prevent soreness. (FND)

■ Asparaginase, an enzyme that inhibits the synthesis of deoxyribonucleic acid and protein, is used to treat acute lymphocytic leukemia. (M-S)

■ To relieve a patient's sore throat that's caused by nasogastric tube irritation, the nurse should provide anesthetic lozenges, as prescribed. (M-S)

■ For the first 12 to 24 hours after gastric surgery, the stomach contents (obtained by suctioning) are brown. (M-S)

■ During gastric lavage, a nasogastric tube is inserted, the stomach is flushed, and ingested substances are removed through the tube. (FND)

■ After gastric suctioning is discontinued, a patient who is recovering from a subtotal gastrectomy should receive a clear liquid diet. (M-S)

■ In documenting drainage on a surgical dressing, the nurse should include the size, color, and consistency of the drainage (for example, "10 mm of brown mucoid drainage noted on dressing"). (FND)

■ Immunization for hepatitis B should be administered at birth, 1 month, and 6 months of age. (PED)

■ The classic signs and symptoms of pyloric stenosis are a palpable olive-sized mass (called a pyloric olive) in the right upper quadrant, strong peristaltic movements from left to right during meals, and projectile vomiting. (PED)

■ The descending colon is the preferred site for a permanent colostomy. (M-S)

■ In rare cases, electroconvulsive therapy causes arrhythmias and death. (PSY)

■ A patient who is scheduled for electroconvulsive therapy should receive nothing by mouth after midnight to prevent aspiration while under anesthesia. (PSY)

Valvular insufficiency in the veins commonly causes varicosity.   (M-S)

A patient with a colostomy should restrict fat and fibrous foods and should avoid foods that can obstruct the stoma, such as corn, nuts, and cabbage.   (M-S)

A patient who is receiving chemotherapy is placed in reverse isolation because the white blood cell count may be depressed.   (M-S)

Symptoms of mitral valve stenosis are caused by improper emptying of the left atrium.   (M-S)

Persistent bleeding after open heart surgery may require the administration of protamine sulfate to reverse the effects of heparin sodium used during surgery.   (M-S)

The nurse should teach a patient with heart failure to take digoxin and other drugs as prescribed, to restrict sodium intake, to restrict fluids as prescribed, to get adequate rest, to increase walking and other activities gradually, to avoid extremes of temperature, to report signs of recurrence, and to keep regular follow-up appointments.   (M-S)

The nurse should check and maintain the patency of all connections for a chest tube. If an air leak is detected, the nurse should place one Kelly clamp near the insertion site. If the bubbling stops, the leak is in the thoracic cavity and the physician should be notified immediately. If the leak continues, the nurse should take a second clamp, work down the tube until the leak is located, and stop the leak.   (M-S)

In two-person cardiopulmonary resuscitation, the rescuers administer 60 chest compressions per minute and 1 breath for every 5 compressions.   (M-S)

Mitral valve stenosis can result from rheumatic fever.   (M-S)

Atelectasis is incomplete expansion of lung segments or lobules (clusters of alveoli). It may cause the lung or lobe to collapse.   (M-S)

The nurse should instruct a patient who has an ileal conduit to empty the collection device frequently because the weight of the urine may cause the device to slip from the skin.   (M-S)

A patient who is receiving cardiopulmonary resuscitation should be placed on a solid, flat surface.   (M-S)

■ Brain damage occurs 4 to 6 minutes after cardiopulmonary function ceases.   (M-S)

■ *Climacteric* is the transition period during which a woman's reproductive function diminishes and gradually disappears.   (M-S)

■ After infratentorial surgery, the patient should remain on his side, flat in bed.   (M-S)

■ To elicit Babinski's reflex, the nurse strokes the sole of the patient's foot with a moderately sharp object, such as a thumbnail.   (FND)

■ A positive Babinski's reflex is shown by dorsiflexion of the great toe and fanning out of the other toes.   (FND)

■ In a patient who has an ulcer, milk is contraindicated because its high calcium content stimulates secretion of gastric acid.   (M-S)

■ When assessing a patient for bladder distention, the nurse should check the contour of the lower abdomen for a rounded mass above the symphysis pubis.   (FND)

■ A patient who has a positive test result for human immunodeficiency virus has been exposed to the virus associated with acquired immunodeficiency syndrome (AIDS), but doesn't necessarily have AIDS.   (M-S)

■ A common complication after prostatectomy is circulatory failure caused by bleeding.   (M-S)

■ In most neonates who are born with human immunodeficiency virus–positive blood, acquired immunodeficiency syndrome develops within 4 months.   (PED)

■ Human immunodeficiency virus (HIV) has been cultured in breast milk and can be transmitted by an HIV-positive mother who breast-feeds her infant.   (MAT)

■ In right-sided heart failure, a major focus of nursing care is decreasing the workload of the heart.   (M-S)

■ Signs and symptoms of digoxin toxicity include nausea, vomiting, confusion, and arrhythmias.   (M-S)

■ The best way to prevent pressure ulcers is to reposition the bedridden patient at least every 2 hours.   (FND)

An asthma attack typically begins with wheezing, coughing, and increasing respiratory distress.   (M-S)

In a patient who is recovering from a tonsillectomy, frequent swallowing suggests hemorrhage.   (M-S)

Ileostomies and Hartmann's colostomies are permanent stomas. Loop colostomies and double-barrel colostomies are temporary ones.   (M-S)

A patient who has an ileostomy should eat foods, such as spinach and parsley, because they act as intestinal tract deodorizers.   (M-S)

An adrenalectomy can decrease steroid production, which can cause extensive loss of sodium and water.   (M-S)

A fever in the first 24 hours postpartum is most likely caused by dehydration rather than infection.   (MAT)

Antiembolism stockings decompress the superficial blood vessels, reducing the risk of thrombus formation.   (FND)

Before administering morphine (Duramorph) to a patient who is suspected of having a myocardial infarction, the nurse should check the patient's respiratory rate. If it's less than 12 breaths/minute, emergency equipment should be readily available for intubation if respiratory depression occurs.   (M-S)

A patient who is recovering from supratentorial surgery is normally allowed out of bed 14 to 48 hours after surgery. A patient who is recovering from infratentorial surgery normally remains on bed rest for 3 to 5 days.   (M-S)

Preterm neonates or neonates who can't maintain a skin temperature of at least 97.6° F (36.4° C) should receive care in an incubator (Isolette) or a radiant warmer. In a radiant warmer, a heat-sensitive probe taped to the neonate's skin activates the heater unit automatically to maintain the desired temperature.   (MAT)

After a patient undergoes a femoral-popliteal bypass graft, the nurse must closely monitor the peripheral pulses distal to the operative site and circulation.   (M-S)

■ After a femoral-popliteal bypass graft, the patient should initially be maintained in a semi-Fowler position to avoid flexion of the graft site. Before discharge, the nurse should instruct the patient to avoid positions that put pressure on the graft site until the next follow-up visit.   (M-S)

■ Of the five senses, hearing is the last to be lost in a patient who is entering a coma.   (M-S)

■ In adults, the most convenient veins for venipuncture are the basilic and median cubital veins in the antecubital space.   (FND)

■ Cholelithiasis causes an enlarged, edematous gallbladder with multiple stones and an elevated bilirubin level.   (M-S)

■ The antiviral agent zidovudine (Retrovir) successfully slows replication of the human immunodeficiency virus, thereby slowing the development of acquired immunodeficiency syndrome.   (M-S)

■ Severe rheumatoid arthritis causes marked edema and congestion, spindle-shaped joints, and severe flexion deformities.   (M-S)

■ A patient with acquired immunodeficiency syndrome should advise his sexual partners of his human immunodeficiency virus status and observe sexual precautions, such as abstinence or condom use.   (M-S)

■ If a radioactive implant becomes dislodged, the nurse should retrieve it with tongs, place it in a lead-shielded container, and notify the radiology department.   (M-S)

■ A patient who is undergoing radiation therapy should pat his skin dry to avoid abrasions that could easily become infected.   (M-S)

■ During radiation therapy, a patient should have frequent blood tests, especially white blood cell and platelet counts.   (M-S)

■ The nurse should administer an aluminum hydroxide antacid at least 1 hour after an enteric-coated drug because it can cause premature release of the enteric-coated drug in the stomach.   (M-S)

■ By age 1, an infant usually has tripled his birth weight and can take steps with support.   (PED)

■ *Acid-base balance* is the body's hydrogen ion concentration, a measure of the ratio of carbonic acid to bicarbonate ions (1 part carbonic acid to 20 parts bicarbonate is normal).   (M-S)

Amyotrophic lateral sclerosis causes progressive atrophy and wasting of muscle groups that eventually affects the respiratory muscles.   (M-S)

Metabolic acidosis is caused by abnormal loss of bicarbonate ions or excessive production or retention of acid ions.   (M-S)

Hemianopsia is defective vision or blindness in one-half of the visual field of one or both eyes.   (M-S)

Systemic lupus erythematosus causes early-morning joint stiffness and facial erythema in a butterfly pattern.   (M-S)

After total knee replacement, the patient should remain in the semi-Fowler position, with the affected leg elevated.   (M-S)

In a patient who is receiving transpyloric feedings, the nurse should watch for dumping syndrome and hypovolemic shock because the stomach is being bypassed.   (M-S)

Two to three hours before beginning a tube feeding, the nurse should aspirate the patient's stomach contents to verify that gastric emptying is adequate.   (FND)

If a total parenteral nutrition infusion must be interrupted, the nurse should administer dextrose 5% in water at a similar rate. Abrupt cessation can cause hypoglycemia.   (M-S)

People with type O blood are considered universal donors.   (FND)

People with type AB blood are considered universal recipients.   (FND)

In setting-sun sign, which reflects prolonged increased intracranial pressure in children, the eyes are forced downward so that a rim of sclera shows above the irises.   (PED)

Status epilepticus is treated with I.V. diazepam (Valium) and phenytoin (Dilantin).   (M-S)

Disequilibrium syndrome causes nausea, vomiting, restlessness, and twitching in patients who are undergoing dialysis. It's caused by a rapid fluid shift.   (M-S)

Electroconvulsive therapy is normally used for patients who have severe depression that doesn't respond to drug therapy.   (PSY)

For electroconvulsive therapy to be effective, the patient usually receives 6 to 12 treatments at a rate of 2 to 3 per week.   (PSY)

An indication that spinal shock is resolving is the return of reflex activity in the arms and legs below the level of injury.   (M-S)

Hypovolemia is the most common and fatal complication of severe acute pancreatitis.   (M-S)

In a patient with stomatitis, oral care includes rinsing the mouth with a mixture of equal parts of hydrogen peroxide and water three times daily.   (M-S)

Hertz (Hz) is the unit of measurement of sound frequency.   (FND)

In otitis media, the tympanic membrane is bright red and lacks its characteristic light reflex (cone of light).   (M-S)

Hearing protection is required when the sound intensity exceeds 84 dB. Double hearing protection is required if it exceeds 104 dB.   (FND)

In patients who have pericardiocentesis, fluid is aspirated from the pericardial sac for analysis or to relieve cardiac tamponade.   (M-S)

During labor, the resting phase between contractions is at least 30 seconds.   (MAT)

Urticaria is an early sign of hemolytic transfusion reaction.   (M-S)

During peritoneal dialysis, a return of brown dialysate suggests bowel perforation. The physician should be notified immediately.   (M-S)

An early sign of ketoacidosis is polyuria, which is caused by osmotic diuresis.   (M-S)

Patients who have multiple sclerosis should visually inspect their extremities to ensure proper alignment and freedom from injury.   (M-S)

A child who has cystic fibrosis should take pancreatic enzyme replacements with meals and snacks.   (PED)

Prothrombin, a clotting factor, is produced in the liver.   (FND)

Aspirated red bone marrow usually appears rust-red, with visible fatty material and white bone fragments.   (M-S)

▨ If a patient is menstruating when a urine sample is collected, the nurse should note this on the laboratory request. **(FND)**

▨ During lumbar puncture, the nurse must note the initial intracranial pressure and the color of the cerebrospinal fluid. **(FND)**

▨ If a patient can't cough to provide a sputum sample for culture, a heated aerosol treatment can be used to help to obtain a sample. **(FND)**

▨ The *Dick test* detects scarlet fever antigens and immunity or susceptibility to scarlet fever. A positive result indicates no immunity; a negative result indicates immunity. **(M-S)**

▨ The *Schick test* detects diphtheria antigens and immunity or susceptibility to diphtheria. A positive result indicates no immunity; a negative result indicates immunity. **(M-S)**

▨ The recommended adult dosage of sucralfate (Carafate) for duodenal ulcer is 1 g (1 tablet) four times daily 1 hour before meals and at bedtime. **(M-S)**

▨ If eye ointment and eyedrops must be instilled in the same eye, the eyedrops should be instilled first. **(FND)**

▨ When leaving an isolation room, the nurse should remove her gloves before her mask because fewer pathogens are on the mask. **(FND)**

▨ *Lochia rubra* is the vaginal discharge of almost pure blood that occurs during the first few days after childbirth. **(MAT)**

▨ *Lochia serosa* is the serous vaginal discharge that occurs 4 to 7 days after childbirth. **(MAT)**

▨ *Lochia alba* is the vaginal discharge of decreased blood and increased leukocytes that's the final stage of lochia. It occurs 7 to 10 days after childbirth. **(MAT)**

▨ A patient with facial burns or smoke or heat inhalation should be admitted to the hospital for 24-hour observation for delayed tracheal edema. **(M-S)**

▨ In addition to patient teaching, preparation for a colostomy includes withholding oral intake overnight, performing bowel preparation, and administering a cleansing enema. **(M-S)**

- Skeletal traction, which is applied to a bone with wire pins or tongs, is the most effective means of traction. (FND)

- The physiologic changes caused by burn injuries can be divided into two stages: the hypovolemic stage, during which intravascular fluid shifts into the interstitial space, and the diuretic stage, during which capillary integrity and intravascular volume are restored, usually 48 to 72 hours after the injury. (M-S)

- The nurse should change total parenteral nutrition tubing every 24 hours and the peripheral I.V. access site dressing every 72 hours. (M-S)

- The total parenteral nutrition solution should be stored in a refrigerator and removed 30 to 60 minutes before use. Delivery of a chilled solution can cause pain, hypothermia, venous spasm, and venous constriction. (FND)

- *Colostrum*, the precursor of milk, is the first secretion from the breasts after delivery. (MAT)

- The length of the uterus increases from 2½" (6.3 cm) before pregnancy to 12½" (32 cm) at term. (MAT)

- To estimate the true conjugate (the smallest inlet measurement of the pelvis), deduct 1.5 cm from the diagonal conjugate (usually 12 cm). A true conjugate of 10.5 cm enables the fetal head (usually 10 cm) to pass. (MAT)

- The smallest outlet measurement of the pelvis is the intertuberous diameter, which is the transverse diameter between the ischial tuberosities. (MAT)

- Electronic fetal monitoring is used to assess fetal well-being during labor. If compromised fetal status is suspected, fetal blood pH may be evaluated by obtaining a scalp sample. (MAT)

- A patient whose carbon monoxide level is 20% to 30% should be treated with 100% humidified oxygen. (M-S)

- When in the room of a patient who is in isolation for tuberculosis, staff and visitors should wear ultrafilter masks. (M-S)

- When providing skin care immediately after pin insertion, the nurse's primary concern is prevention of bone infection. (M-S)

A diagnosis of cystic fibrosis is confirmed by a pilocarpine iontophoresis sweat test. Sodium and chloride concentrations of 50 to 60 mEq/L strongly suggest cystic fibrosis.   (PED)

After an amputation, moist skin may indicate venous stasis; dry skin may indicate arterial obstruction.   (M-S)

Drugs aren't routinely injected intramuscularly into edematous tissue because they may not be absorbed.   (FND)

In a patient who is receiving dialysis, an internal shunt is working if the nurse feels a thrill on palpation or hears a bruit on auscultation. (M-S)

In a patient with viral hepatitis, the parenchymal, or Kupffer's, cells of the liver become severely inflamed, enlarged, and necrotic.   (M-S)

Early signs of acquired immunodeficiency syndrome include fatigue, night sweats, enlarged lymph nodes, anorexia, weight loss, pallor, and fever.   (M-S)

When caring for a patient who has a radioactive implant, health care workers should stay as far away from the radiation source as possible. They should remember the axiom, "If you double the distance, you quarter the dose."   (M-S)

During the manic phase of bipolar affective disorder, nursing care is directed at slowing the patient down because the patient may die as a result of self-induced exhaustion or injury.   (PSY)

For a patient with Alzheimer's disease, the nursing care plan should focus on safety measures.   (PSY)

Growth disturbances, such as bone shortening or overgrowth, may occur in children as a result of a fracture of the epiphyseal plate.   (PED)

In an emergency delivery, enough pressure should be applied to the emerging fetus's head to guide the descent and prevent a rapid change in pressure within the molded fetal skull.   (MAT)

After delivery, a multiparous woman is more susceptible to bleeding than a primiparous woman because her uterine muscles may be overstretched and may not contract efficiently.   (MAT)

A patient who has Parkinson's disease should be instructed to walk with a broad-based gait.   (M-S)

- The cardinal signs of Parkinson's disease are muscle rigidity, a tremor that begins in the fingers, and akinesia.   **(M-S)**

- In a patient with Parkinson's disease, levodopa (Dopar) is prescribed to compensate for the dopamine deficiency.   **(M-S)**

- A patient who has multiple sclerosis is at increased risk for pressure ulcers.   **(M-S)**

- Pill-rolling tremor is a classic sign of Parkinson's disease.   **(M-S)**

- For a patient with Parkinson's disease, nursing interventions are palliative.   **(M-S)**

- Fat embolism, a serious complication of a long-bone fracture, causes fever, tachycardia, tachypnea, and anxiety.   **(M-S)**

- Metrorrhagia (bleeding between menstrual periods) may be the first sign of cervical cancer.   **(M-S)**

- After sexual assault, the patient's needs are the primary concern, followed by medicolegal considerations.   **(PSY)**

- Mannitol is a hypertonic solution and an osmotic diuretic that's used in the treatment of increased intracranial pressure.   **(M-S)**

- When caring for a comatose patient, the nurse should explain each action to the patient in a normal voice.   **(FND)**

- Dentures should be cleaned in a sink that's lined with a washcloth.   **(FND)**

- A patient should void within 8 hours after surgery.   **(FND)**

- An EEG identifies normal and abnormal brain waves.   **(FND)**

- The classic sign of an absence seizure is a vacant facial expression. **(M-S)**

- Migraine headaches cause persistent, severe pain that usually occurs in the temporal region.   **(M-S)**

- A patient who is in a bladder retraining program should be given an opportunity to void every 2 hours during the day and twice at night. **(M-S)**

- In a patient with a head injury, a decrease in level of consciousness is a cardinal sign of increased intracranial pressure.   **(M-S)**

▨ Samples of feces for ova and parasite tests should be delivered to the laboratory without delay and without refrigeration. **(FND)**

▨ The autonomic nervous system regulates the cardiovascular and respiratory systems. **(FND)**

▨ Ergotamine (Ergomar) is most effective when taken during the prodromal phase of a migraine or vascular headache. **(M-S)**

▨ Treatment of acute pancreatitis includes nasogastric suctioning to decompress the stomach and meperidine (Demerol) for pain. **(M-S)**

▨ Symptoms of hiatal hernia include a feeling of fullness in the upper abdomen or chest, heartburn, and pain similar to that of angina pectoris. **(M-S)**

▨ The incidence of cholelithiasis is higher in women who have had children than in any other group. **(M-S)**

▨ Acetaminophen (Tylenol) overdose can severely damage the liver. **(M-S)**

▨ The prominent clinical signs of advanced cirrhosis are ascites and jaundice. **(M-S)**

▨ The first symptom of pancreatitis is steady epigastric pain or left upper quadrant pain that radiates from the umbilical area or the back. **(M-S)**

▨ *Somnambulism* is the medical term for sleepwalking. **(M-S)**

▨ Epinephrine (Adrenalin) is a vasoconstrictor. **(M-S)**

▨ An untreated liver laceration or rupture can progress rapidly to hypovolemic shock. **(M-S)**

▨ *Obstipation* is extreme, intractable constipation caused by an intestinal obstruction. **(M-S)**

▨ When providing tracheostomy care, the nurse should insert the catheter gently into the tracheostomy tube. When withdrawing the catheter, the nurse should apply intermittent suction for no more than 15 seconds and use a slight twisting motion. **(FND)**

▨ A low-residue diet includes such foods as roasted chicken, rice, and pasta. **(FND)**

A rectal tube shouldn't be inserted for longer than 20 minutes because it can irritate the rectal mucosa and cause loss of sphincter control.

(FND)

The definitive test for diagnosing cancer is biopsy with cytologic examination of the specimen. (M-S)

Patients who are in a maintenance program for narcotic abstinence syndrome receive 10 to 40 mg of methadone (Dolophine) in a single daily dose and are monitored to ensure that the drug is ingested. (PSY)

Arthrography requires injection of a contrast medium and can identify joint abnormalities. (M-S)

Brompton's cocktail is prescribed to help relieve pain in patients who have terminal cancer. (M-S)

A patient's bed bath should proceed in this order: face, neck, arms, hands, chest, abdomen, back, legs, perineum. (FND)

To prevent injury when lifting and moving a patient, the nurse should primarily use the upper leg muscles. (FND)

A *sarcoma* is a malignant tumor in connective tissue. (M-S)

Aluminum hydroxide (Amphojel) neutralizes gastric acid. (M-S)

Subluxation is partial dislocation or separation, with spontaneous reduction of a joint. (M-S)

Patient preparation for cholecystography includes ingestion of a contrast medium and a low-fat evening meal. (FND)

Barbiturates can cause confusion and delirium in an elderly patient who has an organic brain disorder. (M-S)

In a patient with arthritis, physical therapy is indicated to promote optimal functioning. (M-S)

Some patients who have hepatitis A may be anicteric (without jaundice) and lack symptoms, but some have headaches, jaundice, anorexia, fatigue, fever, and respiratory tract infection. (M-S)

Hepatitis A is usually mild and won't advance to a carrier state. (M-S)

■ While an occupied bed is being changed, the patient should be covered with a bath blanket to promote warmth and prevent exposure.   (FND)

■ In the preicteric phase of all forms of hepatitis, the patient is highly contagious.   (M-S)

■ Enteric precautions are required for a patient who has hepatitis A. (M-S)

■ Cholecystography is ineffective in a patient who has jaundice as a result of gallbladder disease. The liver cells can't transport the contrast medium to the biliary tract.   (M-S)

■ *Anticipatory grief* is mourning that occurs for an extended time when the patient realizes that death is inevitable.   (FND)

■ In a patient who has diabetes insipidus, dehydration is a concern because diabetes causes polyuria.   (M-S)

■ In a patient who has a reducible hernia, the protruding mass spontaneously retracts into the abdomen.   (M-S)

■ The following foods can alter the color of the feces: beets (red), cocoa (dark red or brown), licorice (black), spinach (green), and meat protein (dark brown).   (FND)

■ Stress management is a short-range goal of psychotherapy.   (PSY)

■ The mood most often experienced by a patient with organic brain syndrome is irritability.   (PSY)

■ Creative intuition is controlled by the right side of the brain.   (PSY)

■ Methohexital (Brevital) is the general anesthetic that's administered to patients who are scheduled for electroconvulsive therapy.   (PSY)

■ When preparing for a skull X-ray, the patient should remove all jewelry and dentures.   (FND)

■ The decision to use restraints should be based on the patient's safety needs.   (PSY)

■ Diphenhydramine (Benadryl) relieves the extrapyramidal adverse effects of psychotropic drugs.   (PSY)

- In a patient who is stabilized on lithium (Eskalith) therapy, blood lithium levels should be checked 8 to 12 hours after the first dose, then two or three times weekly during the first month. Levels should be checked weekly to monthly during maintenance therapy.   **(PSY)**

- To prevent purple glove syndrome, a nurse shouldn't administer I.V. phenytoin (Dilantin) through a vein in the back of the hand, but should use a larger vessel.   **(M-S)**

- The primary purpose of psychotropic drugs is to decrease the patient's symptoms, which improves function and increases compliance with therapy.   **(PSY)**

- *Manipulation* is a maladaptive method of meeting one's needs because it disregards the needs and feelings of others.   **(PSY)**

- If a patient has symptoms of lithium toxicity, the nurse should withhold one dose and call the physician.   **(PSY)**

- A patient who is taking lithium (Eskalith) for bipolar affective disorder must maintain a balanced diet with adequate salt intake.   **(PSY)**

- A patient who constantly seeks approval or assistance from staff members and other patients is demonstrating dependent behavior.   **(PSY)**

- During stage III of surgical anesthesia, unconsciousness occurs and surgery is permitted.   **(M-S)**

- Alcoholics Anonymous advocates total abstinence from alcohol.   **(PSY)**

- Methylphenidate (Ritalin) is the drug of choice for treating attention deficit hyperactivity disorder in children.   **(PSY)**

- Setting limits is the most effective way to control manipulative behavior.   **(PSY)**

- Violent outbursts are common in a patient who has borderline personality disorder.   **(PSY)**

- When working with a depressed patient, the nurse should explore meaningful losses.   **(PSY)**

- An *illusion* is a misinterpretation of an actual environmental stimulus.   **(PSY)**

Anxiety is nonspecific; fear is specific.   **(PSY)**

Extrapyramidal adverse effects are common in patients who take anti-psychotic drugs.   **(PSY)**

The nurse should encourage an angry patient to follow a physical exercise program as one of the ways to ventilate feelings.   **(PSY)**

Depression is clinically significant if it's characterized by exaggerated feelings of sadness, melancholy, dejection, worthlessness, and hopelessness that are inappropriate or out of proportion to reality.   **(PSY)**

Free-floating anxiety is anxiousness with generalized apprehension and pessimism for unknown reasons.   **(PSY)**

In a patient who is experiencing intense anxiety, the fight-or-flight reaction (alarm reflex) may take over.   **(PSY)**

The fight-or-flight response is a sympathetic nervous system response.   **(FND)**

Confabulation is the use of imaginary experiences or made-up information to fill missing gaps of memory.   **(PSY)**

When starting a therapeutic relationship with a patient, the nurse should explain that the purpose of the therapy is to produce a positive change.   **(PSY)**

A basic assumption of psychoanalytic theory is that all behavior has meaning.   **(PSY)**

A 6- to 8-month-old infant should be able to sit without assistance.   **(PED)**

Types of regional anesthesia include spinal, caudal, intercostal, epidural, and brachial plexus.   **(M-S)**

Masturbation is a normal activity in prepubescent children and adolescents.   **(PED)**

The first step in managing drug overdose or drug toxicity is to establish and maintain an airway.   **(M-S)**

Catharsis is the expression of deep feelings and emotions.   **(PSY)**

Respiratory paralysis occurs in stage IV of anesthesia (toxic stage). **(M-S)**

- Neonates who are delivered by cesarean birth have a higher incidence of respiratory distress syndrome.   (MAT)

- The nurse should suggest ambulation to a postpartum patient who has gas pain and flatulence.   (MAT)

- Massaging the uterus helps to stimulate contractions after the placenta is delivered.   (MAT)

- When providing phototherapy to a neonate, the nurse should cover the neonate's eyes and genital area.   (MAT)

- In stage I of anesthesia, the patient is conscious and tranquil.   (M-S)

- Dyspnea and sharp, stabbing pain that increases with respiration are symptoms of pleurisy, which can be a complication of pneumonia or tuberculosis.   (M-S)

- Bronchovesicular breath sounds in peripheral lung fields are abnormal and suggest pneumonia.   (FND)

- *Wheezing* is an abnormal, high-pitched breath sound that's accentuated on expiration.   (FND)

- Wax or a foreign body in the ear should be flushed out gently by irrigation with warm saline solution.   (FND)

- If a patient complains that his hearing aid is "not working," the nurse should check the switch first to see if it's turned on and then check the batteries.   (FND)

- The nurse should grade hyperactive biceps and triceps reflexes as +4.   (FND)

- Vertigo is the major symptom of inner ear infection or disease.   (M-S)

- Loud talking is a sign of hearing impairment.   (M-S)

- A patient who has an upper respiratory tract infection should blow his nose with both nostrils open.   (M-S)

- Infants with sickle cell anemia should receive standard well-baby care, including immunizations.   (PED)

- An infant who has gastroesophageal reflux should receive formula thickened with cereal.   (PED)

A patient who has had a cataract removed can begin most normal activities in 3 or 4 days; however, the patient shouldn't bend and lift until a physician approves these activities. **(M-S)**

If two eye medications are prescribed for twice-daily instillation, they should be administered 5 minutes apart. **(FND)**

Symptoms of corneal transplant rejection include eye irritation and decreasing visual field. **(M-S)**

A child should have a fluoride treatment twice a year. **(PED)**

Wisdom teeth appear between ages 17 and 21. **(PED)**

The narcotic antagonist naloxone (Narcan) may be given to a neonate to correct respiratory depression caused by narcotic administration to the mother during labor. **(MAT)**

In a neonate, symptoms of respiratory distress syndrome include expiratory grunting or whining, sandpaper breath sounds, and seesaw retractions. **(MAT)**

In a postoperative patient, forcing fluids helps prevent constipation. **(FND)**

Cerebral palsy presents as asymmetrical movement, irritability, and excessive, feeble crying in a long, thin infant. **(MAT)**

According to the pleasure principle, the psyche seeks pleasure and avoids unpleasant experiences, regardless of the consequences. **(PSY)**

The nurse should assess a breech-birth neonate for hydrocephalus, hematomas, fractures, and other anomalies caused by birth trauma. **(MAT)**

Children ages 3 to 5 don't conceive of death in final terms, but fear separation from parents. **(PED)**

Children ages 5 to 9 view death as a destructive force or, conversely, as an angel coming in the night. They accept death as a final state, but don't believe that they are targets. **(PED)**

A patient who has a *conversion disorder* resolves a psychological conflict through the loss of a specific physical function (for example, paralysis, blindness, or inability to swallow). This loss of function is involuntary, but diagnostic tests show no organic cause. **(PSY)**

- Graves' disease (hyperthyroidism) is manifested by weight loss, nervousness, dyspnea, palpitations, heat intolerance, increased thirst, exophthalmos (bulging eyes), and goiter. **(M-S)**

- When a patient is admitted to the unit in active labor, the nurse's first action is to listen for fetal heart tones. **(MAT)**

- In a neonate, long, brittle fingernails are a sign of postmaturity. **(MAT)**

- Desquamation (skin peeling) is common in postmature neonates. **(MAT)**

- The four types of lipoprotein are chylomicrons (the lowest-density lipoproteins), very-low-density lipoproteins, low-density lipoproteins, and high-density lipoproteins. Health care professionals use cholesterol level fractionation to assess a patient's risk of coronary artery disease. **(M-S)**

- Greenstick fractures are the most common fractures in children. **(PED)**

- A nurse must provide care in accordance with standards of care established by the American Nurses Association, state regulations, and facility policy. **(FND)**

- The *kilocalorie* (kcal) is a unit of energy measurement that represents the amount of heat needed to raise the temperature of 1 kilogram of water 1° C. **(FND)**

- A child with measles or chickenpox requires respiratory isolation. **(PED)**

- As nutrients move through the body, they undergo ingestion, digestion, absorption, transport, cell metabolism, and excretion. **(FND)**

- The body metabolizes alcohol at a fixed rate, regardless of serum concentration. **(FND)**

- In an alcoholic beverage, proof reflects the percentage of alcohol multiplied by 2. For example, a 100-proof beverage contains 50% alcohol. **(FND)**

- If a patient who is taking amphotericin B (Fungizone) bladder irrigations for a fungal infection has systemic candidiasis and must receive I.V. fluconazole (Diflucan), the irrigations can be discontinued because fluconazole treats the bladder infection as well. **(M-S)**

▨ Patients with adult respiratory distress syndrome can have high peak inspiratory pressures. Therefore, the nurse should monitor these patients closely for signs of spontaneous pneumothorax, such as acute deterioration in oxygenation, absence of breath sounds on the affected side, and crepitus beginning on the affected side. (M-S)

▨ Adverse reactions to cyclosporine (Sandimmune) include renal and hepatic toxicity, central nervous system changes (confusion and delirium), GI bleeding, and hypertension. (M-S)

▨ *Osteoporosis* is a metabolic bone disorder in which the rate of bone resorption exceeds the rate of bone formation. (M-S)

▨ The hallmark of ulcerative colitis is recurrent bloody diarrhea, which commonly contains pus and mucus and alternates with asymptomatic remissions. (M-S)

▨ Safer sexual practices include massaging, hugging, body rubbing, friendly kissing (dry), masturbating, hand-to-genital touching, wearing a condom, and limiting the number of sexual partners. (M-S)

▨ Immunosuppressed patients who contract cytomegalovirus (CMV) are at risk for CMV pneumonia and septicemia, which can be fatal. (M-S)

▨ A *living will* is a witnessed document that states a patient's desire for certain types of care and treatment. These decisions are based on the patient's wishes and views on quality of life. (FND)

▨ The nurse should flush a peripheral heparin lock every 8 hours (if it wasn't used during the previous 8 hours) and as needed with normal saline solution to maintain patency. (FND)

▨ Urinary tract infections can cause urinary urgency and frequency, dysuria, abdominal cramps or bladder spasms, and urethral itching. (M-S)

▨ A mother should allow her infant to breast-feed until the infant is satisfied. The time may vary from 5 to 20 minutes. (MAT)

▨ *Mammography* is a radiographic technique that's used to detect breast cysts or tumors, especially those that aren't palpable on physical examination. (M-S)

▦ To promote early detection of testicular cancer, the nurse should palpate the testes during routine physical examinations and encourage the patient to perform monthly self-examinations during a warm shower.

(M-S)

▦ *Quality assurance* is a method of determining whether nursing actions and practices meet established standards. (FND)

▦ Patients who have thalassemia minor require no treatment. Those with thalassemia major require frequent transfusions of red blood cells.

(M-S)

▦ The five rights of medication administration are the right patient, right drug, right dose, right route of administration, and right time.

(FND)

▦ The *evaluation phase* of the nursing process is to determine whether nursing interventions have enabled the patient to meet the desired goals.

(FND)

▦ Outside of the hospital setting, only the sublingual and translingual forms of nitroglycerin should be used to relieve acute anginal attacks.   (FND)

▦ The *implementation phase* of the nursing process involves recording the patient's response to the nursing plan, putting the nursing plan into action, delegating specific nursing interventions, and coordinating the patient's activities. (FND)

▦ The Patient's Bill of Rights offers patients guidance and protection by stating the responsibilities of the hospital and its staff toward patients and their families during hospitalization. (FND)

▦ To minimize omission and distortion of facts, the nurse should record information as soon as it's gathered. (FND)

▦ When assessing a patient's health history, the nurse should record the current illness chronologically, beginning with the onset of the problem and continuing to the present. (FND)

▦ Chlordiazepoxide (Librium) is the drug of choice for treating alcohol withdrawal symptoms. (PSY)

For a patient who is at risk for alcohol withdrawal, the nurse should assess the pulse rate and blood pressure every 2 hours for the first 12 hours, every 4 hours for the next 24 hours, and every 6 hours thereafter (unless the patient's condition becomes unstable). **(PSY)**

Alcohol detoxification is most successful when carried out in a structured environment by a supportive, nonjudgmental staff. **(PSY)**

A high level of hepatitis B serum marker that persists for 3 months or more after the onset of acute hepatitis B infection suggests chronic hepatitis or carrier status. **(M-S)**

Neurogenic bladder dysfunction is caused by disruption of nerve transmission to the bladder. It may be caused by certain spinal cord injuries, diabetes, or multiple sclerosis. **(M-S)**

The nurse should follow these guidelines when caring for a patient who is experiencing alcohol withdrawal: Maintain a calm environment, keep intrusions to a minimum, speak slowly and calmly, adjust lighting to prevent shadows and glare, call the patient by name, and have a friend or family member stay with the patient, if possible. **(PSY)**

The therapeutic regimen for an alcoholic patient includes folic acid, thiamine, and multivitamin supplements as well as adequate food and fluids. **(PSY)**

A patient who is addicted to opiates (drugs derived from poppy seeds, such as heroin and morphine) typically experiences withdrawal symptoms within 12 hours after the last dose. The most severe symptoms occur within 48 hours and decrease over the next 2 weeks. **(PSY)**

Oxygen and carbon dioxide move between the lungs and the bloodstream by diffusion. **(M-S)**

To grade the severity of dyspnea, the following system is used: grade 1, shortness of breath on mild exertion, such as walking up steps; grade 2, shortness of breath when walking a short distance at a normal pace on level ground; grade 3, shortness of breath with mild daily activity, such as shaving; grade 4, shortness of breath when supine (orthopnea).

(M-S)

A patient with Crohn's disease should consume a diet low in residue, fiber, and fat, and high in calories, proteins, and carbohydrates. The patient also should take vitamin supplements, especially vitamin K. **(M-S)**

▧ A Logan bar is used postoperatively to prevent suture line strain in a child who has had a cleft lip repair.   (PED)

▧ In the three-bottle urine collection method, the patient cleans the meatus and urinates 10 to 15 ml in the first bottle and 15 to 30 ml (midstream) in the second bottle. Then the physician performs prostatic massage, and the patient voids into the third bottle.   (M-S)

▧ Findings in the three-bottle urine collection method are interpreted as follows: pus in the urine (pyuria) in the first bottle indicates anterior urethritis; bacteria in the urine in the second bottle indicate bladder infection; bacteria in the third bottle indicate prostatitis.   (M-S)

▧ Signs and symptoms of aortic stenosis include a loud, rough systolic murmur over the aortic area; exertional dyspnea; fatigue; angina pectoris; arrhythmias; low blood pressure; and emboli.   (M-S)

▧ *Elective surgery* is primarily a matter of choice. It isn't essential to the patient's survival, but it may improve the patient's health, comfort, or self-esteem.   (M-S)

▧ *Required surgery* is recommended by the physician. It may be delayed, but is inevitable.   (M-S)

▧ *Urgent surgery* must be performed within 24 to 48 hours.   (M-S)

▧ *Emergency surgery* must be performed immediately.   (M-S)

▧ Nitrazine paper is used to test the pH of vaginal discharge to determine the presence of amniotic fluid.   (MAT)

▧ Drug administration is a dependent activity. The nurse can administer or withhold a drug only with the physician's permission.   (FND)

▧ About 85% of arterial emboli originate in the heart chambers.   (M-S)

▧ Pulmonary embolism usually results from thrombi dislodged from the leg veins.   (M-S)

▧ A pregnant patient normally gains 2 to 5 lb (1 to 2.5 kg) during the first trimester and slightly less than 1 lb (0.5 kg) per week during the last two trimesters.   (MAT)

▧ A nurse shouldn't give false assurance to a patient.   (FND)

Neonatal jaundice in the first 24 hours after birth is known as pathological jaundice and is a sign of erythroblastosis fetalis.   (MAT)

A classic difference between abruptio placentae and placenta previa is the degree of pain. Abruptio placentae causes pain, whereas placenta previa causes painless bleeding.   (MAT)

After receiving preoperative medication, a patient isn't competent to sign an informed consent form.   (FND)

The conscious interpretation of pain occurs in the cerebral cortex. (M-S)

To avoid interfering with new cell growth, the dressing on a donor skin graft site shouldn't be disturbed.   (M-S)

A sequela is any abnormal condition that follows and is the result of a disease, a treatment, or an injury.   (M-S)

During sickle cell crisis, patient care includes bed rest, oxygen therapy, analgesics as prescribed, I.V. fluid monitoring, and thorough documentation of fluid intake and output.   (M-S)

Reactive depression is a response to a specific life event.   (PSY)

A patient who has an ileal conduit should maintain a daily fluid intake of 2,000 ml.   (M-S)

The lower central incisors erupt first in an infant, at approximately age 4 to 6 months.   (PED)

In a closed chest drainage system, continuous bubbling in the water seal chamber or bottle indicates a leak.   (M-S)

Palpitation is a sensation of heart pounding or racing associated with normal emotional responses and certain heart disorders.   (M-S)

Fat embolism is likely to occur within the first 24 hours after a long-bone fracture.   (M-S)

Footdrop can occur in a patient with a pelvic fracture as a result of peroneal nerve compression against the head of the fibula.   (M-S)

To promote venous return after an amputation, the nurse should wrap an elastic bandage around the distal end of the stump.   (M-S)

▧ Because a major role of the placenta is to function as a fetal lung, any condition that interrupts normal blood flow to or from the placenta increases fetal partial pressure of arterial carbon dioxide and decreases fetal pH. **(MAT)**

▧ Water that accumulates in the tubing of a ventilator should be removed. **(M-S)**

▧ Precipitate labor lasts for approximately 3 hours and ends with delivery of the neonate. **(MAT)**

▧ Methylergonovine (Methergine) is an oxytocic agent used to prevent and treat postpartum hemorrhage caused by uterine atony or subinvolution. **(MAT)**

▧ As emergency treatment for excessive uterine bleeding, 0.2 mg of methylergonovine (Methergine) is injected I.V. over 1 minute while the patient's blood pressure and uterine contractions are monitored. **(MAT)**

▧ If a child with a febrile illness is scheduled for an immunization, the immunization should be postponed. **(PED)**

▧ Toilet training should begin when a child shows signs of readiness, such as staying dry for 2 hours or longer and verbalizing the urge to urinate. **(PED)**

▧ Most children achieve daytime bladder and bowel control between ages 2 and 3. Failure to achieve toilet training by age 5 doesn't usually indicate pathology, but should be investigated by a physician. **(PED)**

▧ *Projection* is the unconscious assigning of a thought, feeling, or action to someone or something else. **(PSY)**

▧ *Sublimation* is the channeling of unacceptable impulses into socially acceptable behavior. **(PSY)**

▧ *Repression* is an unconscious defense mechanism whereby unacceptable or painful thoughts, impulses, memories, or feelings are pushed from the consciousness or forgotten. **(PSY)**

▧ The most common route for the administration of epinephrine to a patient who is having a severe allergic reaction is the subcutaneous route. **(M-S)**

Hypochondriasis is morbid anxiety about one's health associated with various symptoms that aren't caused by organic disease.　**(PSY)**

Denial is a refusal to acknowledge feelings, thoughts, desires, impulses, or external facts that are consciously intolerable.　**(PSY)**

Reaction formation is the avoidance of anxiety through behavior and attitudes that are the opposite of repressed impulses and drives.　**(PSY)**

Displacement is the transfer of unacceptable feelings to a more acceptable object.　**(PSY)**

Regression is a retreat to an earlier developmental stage.　**(PSY)**

The nurse should use Fowler's position for a patient who has abdominal pain caused by appendicitis.　**(M-S)**

The nurse shouldn't give analgesics to a patient who has abdominal pain caused by appendicitis because these drugs may mask the pain that accompanies a ruptured appendix.　**(M-S)**

As a last-ditch effort, a barbiturate coma may be induced to reverse unrelenting increased intracranial pressure (ICP), which is defined as acute ICP of greater than 40 mm Hg, persistent elevation of ICP above 20 mm Hg, or rapidly deteriorating neurologic status.　**(M-S)**

The primary signs and symptoms of epiglottiditis are stridor and progressive difficulty in swallowing.　**(M-S)**

Salivation is the first step in the digestion of starch.　**(M-S)**

Braxton Hicks contractions are usually felt in the abdomen and don't cause cervical change. True labor contractions are felt in the front of the abdomen and back and lead to progressive cervical dilation and effacement.　**(MAT)**

The average birth weight of neonates born to mothers who smoke is 6 oz (170 g) less than that of neonates born to nonsmoking mothers.　**(MAT)**

When performing cardiopulmonary resuscitation on an infant, the administrator should compress the sternum ½″ to 1″ (1 to 2.5 cm), using two fingers.　**(PED)**

A patient who has a demand pacemaker should measure the pulse rate before rising in the morning, notify the physician if the pulse rate drops by 5 beats/minute, obtain a medical identification card and bracelet, and resume normal activities, including sexual activity.   **(M-S)**

Ventricular septal defect occurs when the septum between the left and right ventricles does not close during the first 8 weeks of gestation.   **(PED)**

Transverse, or loop, colostomy is a temporary procedure that's performed to divert the fecal stream in a patient who has acute intestinal obstruction.   **(M-S)**

According to Erikson, an older adult (age 65 or older) is in the developmental stage of integrity versus despair.   **(PSY)**

Family therapy focuses on the family as a whole rather than the individual. Its major objective is to reestablish rational communication between family members.   **(PSY)**

When lifting a patient, a nurse uses the weight of her body instead of the strength in her arms.   **(FND)**

Normal values for erythrocyte sedimentation rate are 0 to 15 mm/hour for men younger than age 50 and 0 to 20 mm/hour for women younger than age 50.   **(M-S)**

A CK-MB level that's more than 5% of total CK or more than 10 U/L suggests a myocardial infarction.   **(M-S)**

Culdoscopy is visualization of the pelvic organs through the posterior vaginal fornix.   **(MAT)**

Propranolol (Inderal) blocks sympathetic nerve stimuli that increase cardiac work during exercise or stress, which reduces heart rate, blood pressure, and myocardial oxygen consumption.   **(M-S)**

After a myocardial infarction, electrocardiogram changes (ST-segment elevation, T-wave inversion, and Q-wave enlargement) usually appear in the first 24 hours, but may not appear until the 5th or 6th day.   **(M-S)**

Cardiogenic shock is manifested by systolic blood pressure of less than 80 mm Hg, gray skin, diaphoresis, cyanosis, weak pulse rate, tachycardia or bradycardia, and oliguria (less than 30 ml of urine per hour).   **(M-S)**

A patient who is receiving a low-sodium diet shouldn't eat cottage cheese, fish, canned beans, chuck steak, chocolate pudding, Italian salad dressing, dill pickles, and beef broth. **(M-S)**

High-potassium foods include dried prunes, watermelon (15.3 mEq/portion), dried lima beans (14.5 mEq/portion), soybeans, bananas, and oranges. **(M-S)**

A nurse may clarify a physician's explanation about an operation or a procedure to a patient, but must refer questions about informed consent to the physician. **(FND)**

When caring for a patient who is hostile or angry, the nurse should attempt to remain calm, listen impartially, use short sentences, and speak in a firm, quiet voice. **(PSY)**

A sick or injured child who has limited communication skills may be able to express his feelings or concerns by drawing a picture with crayons or markers. **(PED)**

When obtaining a health history from an acutely ill or agitated patient, the nurse should limit questions to those that provide necessary information. **(FND)**

If a chest drainage system line is broken or interrupted, the nurse should clamp the tube immediately. **(FND)**

The nurse shouldn't use her thumb to take a patient's pulse rate because the thumb has a pulse that may be confused with the patient's pulse. **(FND)**

An inspiration and an expiration count as one respiration. **(FND)**

Kussmaul's respirations are faster and deeper than normal respirations and occur without pauses, as in diabetic ketoacidosis. **(M-S)**

Cheyne-Stokes respirations are characterized by alternating periods of apnea and deep, rapid breathing. They occur in patients with central nervous system disorders. **(M-S)**

Hyperventilation can result from an increased frequency of breathing, an increased tidal volume, or both. **(M-S)**

Apnea is the absence of spontaneous respirations. **(M-S)**

▨ Before a thyroidectomy, a patient may receive potassium iodide, anti-thyroid drugs, and propranolol (Inderal) to prevent thyroid storm during surgery. **(M-S)**

▨ *Eupnea* is normal respiration. **(FND)**

▨ During blood pressure measurement, the patient should rest the arm against a surface. Using muscle strength to hold up the arm may raise the blood pressure. **(FND)**

▨ Major, unalterable risk factors for coronary artery disease include heredity, sex, race, and age. **(FND)**

▨ The nurse should teach a pregnant vegetarian to obtain protein from alternative sources, such as nuts, soybeans, and legumes. **(MAT)**

▨ *Inspection* is the most frequently used assessment technique. **(FND)**

▨ The nurse should instruct a pregnant patient to take only prescribed prenatal vitamins because over-the-counter high-potency vitamins may harm the fetus. **(MAT)**

▨ High-sodium foods can cause fluid retention, especially in pregnant patients. **(MAT)**

▨ A pregnant patient can avoid constipation and hemorrhoids by adding fiber to her diet. **(MAT)**

▨ The normal life span of red blood cells (erythrocytes) is 110 to 120 days. **(M-S)**

▨ Ritualism and negativism are typical toddler behaviors. They occur during the developmental stage identified by Erikson as autonomy versus shame and doubt. **(PSY)**

▨ Accidents are the leading cause of death in children and are commonly age-related. For example, toddlers are injured in falls and teenagers are injured in sports. **(PED)**

▨ Urinary tract infections are more common in girls and women than in boys and men because the shorter urethra in the female urinary tract makes the bladder more accessible to bacteria, especially *Escherichia coli*. **(M-S)**

■ Visual acuity of 20/100 means that the patient sees at 20' (6 m) what a person with normal vision sees at 100' (30 m). (M-S)

■ According to Freud, the oral stage occurs between birth and age 18 months. (PED)

■ Penicillin is administered orally 1 to 2 hours before meals or 2 to 3 hours after meals because food may interfere with the drug's absorption. (M-S)

■ For an infant, the nurse should start an I.V. line in a peripheral vein or a vein in the temporal region. (PED)

■ Mild reactions to local anesthetics may include palpitations, tinnitus, vertigo, apprehension, confusion, and a metallic taste in the mouth. (M-S)

■ When administering an oral medication to a toddler, the nurse should have the child place the medication on the back of his tongue and swallow it with fruit juice or water. (PED)

■ Family members of an elderly person in a long-term care facility should transfer some personal items (such as photographs, a favorite chair, and knickknacks) to the person's room to provide a comfortable atmosphere. (FND)

■ About 22% of cardiac output goes to the kidneys. (M-S)

■ To ensure accurate central venous pressure readings, the nurse should place the manometer or transducer level with the phlebostatic axis. (M-S)

■ A patient who has lost 2,000 to 2,500 ml of blood will have a pulse rate of 140 beats/minute (or higher), display a systolic blood pressure of 50 to 60 mm Hg, and appear confused and lethargic. (M-S)

■ Arterial blood is bright red, flows rapidly, and (because it's pumped directly from the heart) spurts with each heartbeat. (M-S)

■ Venous blood is dark red and tends to ooze from a wound. (M-S)

■ Orthostatic blood pressure is taken with the patient in the supine, sitting, and standing positions, with 1 minute between each reading. A 10-mm Hg decrease in blood pressure or an increase in pulse rate of 10 beats/minute suggests volume depletion. (M-S)

■ *Pulsus alternans* is a regular pulse rhythm with alternating weak and strong beats. It occurs in ventricular enlargement because the stroke volume varies with each heartbeat. **(FND)**

■ A pneumatic antishock garment should be used cautiously in pregnant women and patients with head injuries. **(M-S)**

■ After a patient's circulating volume is restored, the nurse should remove the pneumatic antishock garment gradually, starting with the abdominal chamber and followed by each leg. The garment should be removed under a physician's supervision. **(M-S)**

■ Most hemolytic transfusion reactions associated with mismatching of ABO blood types stem from identification number errors. **(M-S)**

■ *Circumstantiality* is a disturbance in associated thought and speech patterns in which a patient gives unnecessary, minute details and digresses into inappropriate thoughts that delay communication of central ideas and goal achievement. **(PSY)**

■ Warming of blood to more than 107° F (41.7° C) can cause hemolysis. **(M-S)**

■ *Cardiac output* is the amount of blood ejected from the heart each minute. It's expressed in liters per minute. **(M-S)**

■ *Stroke volume* is the volume of blood ejected from the heart during systole. **(M-S)**

■ Total parenteral nutrition solution contains dextrose, amino acids, and additives, such as electrolytes, minerals, and vitamins. **(M-S)**

■ The most common type of neurogenic shock is spinal shock. It usually occurs 30 to 60 minutes after a spinal cord injury. **(M-S)**

■ After a spinal cord injury, peristalsis stops within 24 hours and usually returns within 3 to 4 days. **(M-S)**

■ Toxic shock syndrome is manifested by a temperature of at least 102° F (38.8° C), an erythematous rash, and systolic blood pressure of less than 90 mm Hg. From 1 to 2 weeks after the onset of these signs, desquamation (especially on the palms and soles) occurs. **(M-S)**

■ The signs and symptoms of anaphylaxis are commonly caused by histamine release. **(M-S)**

▓ The most common cause of septic shock is gram-negative bacteria, such as *Escherichia coli*, *Klebsiella*, and *Pseudomonas* organisms. **(M-S)**

▓ *Bruits* are vascular sounds that resemble heart murmurs and result from turbulent blood flow through a diseased or partially obstructed artery. **(M-S)**

▓ Urine pH is normally 4.5 to 8.0. **(M-S)**

▓ Urine pH of greater than 8.0 can result from a urinary tract infection, a high-alkali diet, or systemic alkalosis. **(M-S)**

▓ Urine pH of less than 4.5 may be caused by a high-protein diet, fever, or metabolic acidosis. **(M-S)**

▓ Before a percutaneous renal biopsy, the patient should be placed on a firm surface and positioned on the abdomen. A sandbag is placed under the abdomen to stabilize the kidneys. **(M-S)**

▓ Nephrotic syndrome is characterized by marked proteinuria, hypoalbuminemia, mild to severe dependent edema, ascites, and weight gain. **(M-S)**

▓ Underwater exercise is a form of therapy performed in a Hubbard tank. **(M-S)**

▓ Most women with trichomoniasis have a malodorous, frothy, greenish gray vaginal discharge. Other women may have no signs or symptoms. **(M-S)**

▓ Voiding cystourethrography may be performed to detect bladder and urethral abnormalities. Contrast medium is instilled by gentle syringe pressure through a urethral catheter, and overhead X-ray films are taken to visualize bladder filling and excretion. **(M-S)**

▓ Cystourethrography may be performed to identify the cause of urinary tract infections, congenital anomalies, and incontinence. It also is used to assess for prostate lobe hypertrophy in men. **(M-S)**

▓ Herpes simplex is characterized by recurrent episodes of blisters on the skin and mucous membranes. It has two variations. In Type 1, the blisters appear in the nasolabial region; in Type 2, they appear on the genitals, anus, buttocks, and thighs. **(M-S)**

- Most patients with *Chlamydia trachomatis* infection are asymptomatic, but some have an inflamed urethral meatus, dysuria, and urinary urgency and frequency.   (M-S)

- The hypothalamus regulates the autonomic nervous system and endocrine functions.   (M-S)

- If a fetus has late decelerations (a sign of fetal hypoxia), the nurse should instruct the mother to lie on her left side and then administer 8 to 10 L of oxygen per minute by mask or cannula. The nurse should notify the physician. The side-lying position removes pressure on the inferior vena cava.   (MAT)

- Oxytocin (Pitocin) promotes lactation and uterine contractions. (MAT)

- The upper respiratory tract warms and humidifies inspired air and plays a role in taste, smell, and mastication.   (FND)

- A patient whose chest excursion is less than normal (3" to 6" [7.5 to 15 cm]) must use accessory muscles to breathe.   (M-S)

- Signs of accessory muscle use include shoulder elevation, intercostal muscle retraction, and scalene and sternocleidomastoid muscle use during respiration.   (FND)

- Lanugo covers the fetus's body until about 20 weeks' gestation. Then it begins to disappear from the face, trunk, arms, and legs, in that order.   (MAT)

- Although a cleft palate can be repaired at any time, the optimal time for corrective surgery is before the child begins speaking and learns faulty speech habits.   (PED)

- In a neonate, hypoglycemia causes temperature instability, hypotonia, jitteriness, and seizures. Premature, postmature, small-for-gestational-age, and large-for-gestational-age neonates are susceptible to this disorder.   (MAT)

- An infant with a gastrostomy tube should receive a pacifier during feeding unless contraindicated to provide normal sucking activity and satisfy oral needs.   (PED)

- Signs and symptoms of toxicity from thyroid replacement therapy include rapid pulse rate, diaphoresis, irritability, weight loss, dysuria, and sleep disturbance.   (M-S)

The most common allergic reaction to penicillin is a rash.   **(M-S)**

An early sign of aspirin toxicity is deep, rapid respirations.   **(M-S)**

The most serious and irreversible consequence of lead poisoning is mental retardation, which results from neurologic damage.   **(M-S)**

Treatment for Legg-Calvé-Perthes disease consists of restricting weight bearing and using a device, such as an abduction brace or a harness sling, to protect the affected joint while revascularization and bone healing occur.   **(PED)**

To assess dehydration in the adult, the nurse should check skin turgor on the sternum.   **(M-S)**

Legg-Calvé-Perthes disease, or coxa plana, is manifested in aseptic necrosis of the head of the femur.   **(PED)**

For a patient with a peptic ulcer, the type of diet is less important than including foods in the diet that the patient can tolerate.   **(M-S)**

A patient with a colostomy must establish an irrigation schedule so that regular emptying of the bowel occurs without stomal discharge between irrigations.   **(M-S)**

Idea of reference is an incorrect belief that the statements or actions of others are related to oneself.   **(PSY)**

When using rotating tourniquets, the nurse shouldn't restrict the blood supply to an arm or leg for more than 45 minutes at a time.   **(M-S)**

A patient with diabetes should eat high-fiber foods because they blunt the rise in glucose level that normally follows a meal.   **(M-S)**

Jugular vein distention occurs in patients with heart failure because the left ventricle can't empty the heart of blood as fast as blood enters from the right ventricle, resulting in congestion in the entire venous system.   **(M-S)**

When patients use axillary crutches, their palms should bear the brunt of the weight.   **(FND)**

The leading causes of blindness in the United States are diabetes mellitus and glaucoma.   **(M-S)**

■ After a thyroidectomy, the patient should remain in the semi-Fowler position, with his head neither hyperextended nor hyperflexed, to avoid pressure on the suture line. This position can be achieved with the use of a cervical pillow. **(M-S)**

■ Premenstrual syndrome may cause abdominal distention, engorged and painful breasts, backache, headache, nervousness, irritability, restlessness, and tremors. **(M-S)**

■ Treatment of dehiscence (pathologic opening of a wound) consists of covering the wound with a moist sterile dressing and notifying the physician. **(M-S)**

■ When a patient has a radical mastectomy, the ovaries also may be removed because they are a source of estrogen, which stimulates tumor growth. **(M-S)**

■ Atropine blocks the effects of acetylcholine, thereby obstructing its vagal effects on the sinoatrial node and increasing heart rate. **(M-S)**

■ Activities of daily living include eating, bathing, dressing, grooming, toileting, and interacting socially. **(FND)**

■ Salicylates, particularly aspirin, are the treatment of choice in rheumatoid arthritis because they decrease inflammation and relieve joint pain. **(M-S)**

■ Deep, intense pain that usually worsens at night and is unrelated to movement suggests bone pain. **(M-S)**

■ Pain that follows prolonged or excessive exercise and subsides with rest suggests muscle pain. **(M-S)**

■ Normal gait has two phases: the stance phase, in which the patient's foot rests on the ground, and the swing phase, in which the patient's foot moves forward. **(FND)**

■ The major hemodynamic changes associated with cardiogenic shock are decreased left ventricular function and decreased cardiac output. **(M-S)**

■ Before thyroidectomy, the patient should be advised that he may experience hoarseness or loss of his voice for several days after surgery. **(M-S)**

■ Acceptable adverse effects of long-term steroid use include weight gain, acne, headaches, fatigue, and increased urine retention. **(M-S)**

■ Unacceptable adverse effects of long-term steroid use are dizziness on rising, nausea, vomiting, thirst, and pain.   (M-S)

■ After a craniotomy, nursing care includes maintaining normal intracranial pressure, maintaining cerebral perfusion pressure, and preventing injury related to cerebral and cellular ischemia.   (M-S)

■ Neonates typically need to consume 50 to 55 cal per pound of body weight daily.   (MAT)

■ Folic acid and vitamin B_{12} are essential for nucleoprotein synthesis and red blood cell maturation.   (M-S)

■ Immediately after intracranial surgery, nursing care includes not giving the patient anything by mouth until the gag and cough reflexes return, monitoring vital signs and assessing the level of consciousness (LOC) for signs of increasing intracranial pressure, and administering analgesics that don't mask the LOC.   (M-S)

■ Chest physiotherapy includes postural drainage, chest percussion and vibration, and coughing and deep-breathing exercises.   (M-S)

■ The nurse should encourage parents to communicate with their hearing-impaired child through mime, gestures, and body language.   (PED)

■ Kawasaki disease is characterized by a high temperature for 5 days or longer; strawberry tongue; red, dry lips; cervical lymphadenopathy; carditis; edema of the hands; rash on the soles or palms; and bilateral congestion of the ocular conjunctivae.   (PED)

■ Cushing's syndrome results from excessive levels of adrenocortical hormones and is manifested by fat pads on the face (moon face) and over the upper back (buffalo hump), acne, mood swings, hirsutism, amenorrhea, and decreased libido.   (M-S)

■ To prevent an addisonian crisis when discontinuing long-term prednisone (Deltasone) therapy, the nurse should taper the dose slowly to allow for monitoring of disease flare-ups and for the return of hypothalamic-pituitary-adrenal function.   (M-S)

■ *Pulsus paradoxus* is a pulse that becomes weak during inspiration and strong during expiration. It may be a sign of cardiac tamponade. (M-S)

▨ Substances that are expelled through portals of exit include saliva, mucus, feces, urine, vomitus, blood, and vaginal and penile discharges.

(M-S)

▨ A microorganism may be transmitted directly, by contact with an infected body or droplets, or indirectly, by contact with contaminated air, soil, water, or fluids. (M-S)

▨ A postmenopausal woman who receives estrogen therapy is at an increased risk for gallbladder disease and breast cancer. (M-S)

▨ The approximate oxygen concentrations delivered by a nasal cannula are as follows:
1 L = 24%, 2 L = 28%, 3 L = 32%, 4 L= 36%, and 5 L = 40%. (M-S)

▨ Because oxytocin (Pitocin) stimulates powerful uterine contractions during labor, it must be administered under close observation to help prevent maternal and fetal distress. (MAT)

▨ Cardinal features of diabetes insipidus include polydipsia (excessive thirst) and polyuria (increased urination to 5 L/24 hours). (M-S)

▨ A patient with low specific gravity (1.001 to 1.005) may have an increased desire for cold water. (M-S)

▨ Diabetic coma can occur when the blood glucose level drops below 60 mg/dl. (M-S)

▨ For a patient with heart failure, the nurse should elevate the head of the bed 8″ to 12″ (20 to 30 cm), provide a bedside commode, and administer cardiac glycosides and diuretics as prescribed. (M-S)

▨ Group therapy provides an opportunity for each group member to examine interactions, learn and practice successful interpersonal communication skills, and explore emotional conflicts. (PSY)

▨ The primary reason to treat streptococcal sore throat with antibiotics is to protect the heart valves and prevent rheumatic fever. (M-S)

▨ A patient with a nasal fracture may lose consciousness during reduction.

(M-S)

▨ Hoarseness and change in the voice are commonly the first signs of laryngeal cancer. (M-S)

■ The lungs, colon, and rectum are among the most common cancer sites. (M-S)

■ The most common preoperative problem in elderly patients is lower-than-normal total blood volume. (M-S)

■ Mannitol (Osmitrol), an osmotic diuretic, is administered to reduce intraocular or intracranial pressure. (M-S)

■ When a stroke is suspected, the nurse should place the patient on the affected side to promote lung expansion on the unaffected side. (M-S)

■ For a patient who has had chest surgery, the nurse should recommend sitting upright and performing coughing and deep-breathing exercises. These actions promote expansion of the lungs, removal of secretions, and optimal pulmonary functioning. (M-S)

■ During fetal heart rate monitoring, variable decelerations indicate compression or prolapse of the umbilical cord. (MAT)

■ During every sleep cycle, the sleeper passes through four stages of non-rapid-eye-movement sleep and one stage of rapid-eye-movement sleep. (M-S)

■ The phases of mitosis are prophase, metaphase, anaphase, and telophase. (FND)

■ Korsakoff's syndrome is believed to be a chronic form of Wernicke's encephalopathy. It's marked by hallucinations, confabulation, amnesia, and disturbances of orientation. (PSY)

■ A patient who is taking calcifediol (Calderol) should avoid concomitant use of preparations that contain vitamin D. (M-S)

■ A patient should begin and end a 24-hour urine collection period with an empty bladder. For example, if the physician orders urine to be collected from 0800 Thursday to 0800 Friday, the urine voided at 0800 Thursday should be discarded and the urine voided at 0800 Friday should be retained. (M-S)

■ In a patient who is receiving digoxin (Lanoxin), a low potassium level increases the risk of digoxin toxicity. (M-S)

■ Blood urea nitrogen values normally range from 10 to 20 mg/dl. (M-S)

■ Flurazepam (Dalmane) toxicity is manifested by confusion, hallucinations, and ataxia. (M-S)

■ A silent myocardial infarction is one that has no symptoms. (M-S)

■ Adverse reactions to verapamil (Isoptin) include dizziness, headache, constipation, hypotension, and atrioventricular conduction disturbances. The drug also may increase the serum digoxin level. (M-S)

■ When a rectal tube is used to relieve flatulence or enhance peristalsis, it should be inserted for no longer than 20 minutes. (M-S)

■ Yellowish green discharge on a wound dressing indicates infection and should be cultured. (M-S)

■ Sickle cell crisis can cause severe abdominal, thoracic, muscular, and bone pain along with painful swelling of soft tissue in the hands and feet. (M-S)

■ Oral candidiasis (thrush) is characterized by cream-colored or bluish white patches on the oral mucous membrane. (M-S)

■ Treatment for a patient with cystic fibrosis may include drug therapy, exercises to improve breathing and posture, exercises to facilitate mobilization of pulmonary secretions, a high-salt diet, and pancreatic enzyme supplements with snacks and meals. (M-S)

■ After surgical reconstruction of an imperforate anus and formation of a temporary colostomy, an infant should remain prone, with the hips elevated. (PED)

■ A patient with antisocial personality disorder often engages in confrontations with authority figures, such as police, parents, and school officials. (PSY)

■ A patient with paranoid personality disorder exhibits suspicion, hypervigilance, and hostility toward others. (PSY)

■ *Child neglect* is abandonment or failure to provide a safe, secure environment for a child. (PED)

■ Depression is the most common psychiatric disorder. (PSY)

■ Cytomegalovirus is the leading cause of congenital viral infection. (MAT)

■ Most infants with cerebral palsy are long and thin, move asymmetrically, have difficulty feeding, and cry excessively or feebly.   **(PED)**

■ Pancreatic cancer may cause weight loss, jaundice, and intermittent dull-to-severe epigastric pain.   **(M-S)**

■ Adverse reactions to tricyclic antidepressant drugs include tachycardia, orthostatic hypotension, hypomania, lowered seizure threshold, tremors, weight gain, problems with erections or orgasms, and anxiety.   **(PSY)**

■ The nurse should follow standard precautions in the routine care of all patients.   **(FND)**

■ *Metastasis* is the spread of cancer from one organ or body part to another through the lymphatic system, circulation system, or cerebrospinal fluid.   **(M-S)**

■ Tocolytic therapy is indicated in premature labor, but contraindicated in fetal death, fetal distress, or severe hemorrhage.   **(MAT)**

■ The management of pulmonary edema focuses on opening the airways, supporting ventilation and perfusion, improving cardiac functioning, reducing preload, and reducing patient anxiety.   **(M-S)**

■ Factors that contribute to the death of patients with Alzheimer's disease include infection, malnutrition, and dehydration.   **(M-S)**

■ Hodgkin's disease is characterized by painless, progressive enlargement of cervical lymph nodes and other lymphoid tissue as a result of proliferation of Reed-Sternberg cells, histiocytes, and eosinophils.   **(M-S)**

■ Huntington's disease (chorea) is a hereditary disease characterized by degeneration in the cerebral cortex and basal ganglia.   **(M-S)**

■ A patient with Huntington's disease may exhibit suicidal ideation.   **(M-S)**

■ At discharge, an amputee should be able to demonstrate proper stump care and perform stump-toughening exercises.   **(M-S)**

■ Acute tubular necrosis is the most common cause of acute renal failure.   **(M-S)**

■ Common complications of ice water lavage are vomiting and aspiration.   **(M-S)**

■ Foods high in vitamin D include fortified milk, fish, liver, liver oil, herring, and egg yolk. (M-S)

■ Through ultrasonography, the biophysical profile assesses fetal well-being by measuring fetal breathing movements, gross body movements, fetal tone, reactive fetal heart rate (nonstress test), and qualitative amniotic fluid volume. (MAT)

■ For a pelvic examination, the patient should be in the lithotomy position, with the buttocks extending 2½" (6.4 cm) past the end of the examination table. (M-S)

■ If a patient can't assume the lithotomy position for a pelvic examination, she may lie on her left side. (M-S)

■ A male examiner should have a female assistant present during a vaginal examination for the patient's emotional comfort and the examiner's legal protection. (M-S)

■ Cervical secretions are clear and stretchy before ovulation and white and opaque after ovulation. They're normally odorless and don't irritate the mucosa. (M-S)

■ A neonate whose mother has diabetes should be assessed for hyperinsulinism. (MAT)

■ In a patient with preeclampsia, epigastric pain is a late symptom and requires immediate medical intervention. (MAT)

■ After a stillbirth, the mother should be allowed to hold the neonate to help her come to terms with the death. (MAT)

■ The concept of object permanence develops between ages 6 and 8 months. (PED)

■ A child begins to understand cause-and-effect relations at age 2, during the sensorimotor stage. (PED)

■ Attention deficit hyperactivity disorder and learning disabilities are more common among boys than girls. (PED)

■ A patient with an ileostomy shouldn't eat corn because it may obstruct the opening of the pouch. (M-S)

Molding is the process by which the fetal head changes shape to facilitate movement through the birth canal. (MAT)

Liver dysfunction affects the metabolism of certain drugs. (M-S)

If a woman receives a spinal block before delivery, the nurse should monitor the patient's blood pressure closely. (MAT)

If a woman suddenly becomes hypotensive during labor, the nurse should increase the infusion rate of I.V. fluids as prescribed. (MAT)

The best technique for assessing jaundice in a neonate is to blanch the tip of the nose or the area just above the umbilicus. (MAT)

During fetal heart monitoring, early deceleration is caused by compression of the head during labor. (MAT)

After the placenta is delivered, the nurse may add oxytocin (Pitocin) to the patient's I.V. solution, as prescribed, to promote postpartum involution of the uterus and stimulate lactation. (MAT)

Pica is a craving to eat nonfood items, such as dirt, crayons, chalk, glue, starch, or hair. It may occur during pregnancy and can endanger the fetus. (MAT)

A pregnant patient should take folic acid because this nutrient is required for rapid cell division. (MAT)

Edema that accompanies burns and malnutrition is caused by decreased osmotic pressure in the capillaries. (M-S)

Hyponatremia is most likely to occur as a complication of nasogastric suctioning. (M-S)

In a man who has complete spinal cord separation at S4, erection and ejaculation aren't possible. (M-S)

The early signs of pulmonary edema (dyspnea on exertion and coughing) reflect interstitial fluid accumulation and decreased ventilation and alveolar perfusion. (M-S)

Methylprednisolone (Solu-Medrol) is a first-line drug used to control edema after spinal cord trauma. (M-S)

For the patient who is recovering from an intracranial bleed, the nurse should maintain a quiet, restful environment for the first few days. **(M-S)**

A woman who is taking clomiphene (Clomid) to induce ovulation should be informed of the possibility of multiple births with this drug. **(MAT)**

Neurosyphilis is associated with widespread damage to the central nervous system, including general paresis, personality changes, slapping gait, and blindness. **(M-S)**

A woman who has had a spinal cord injury can still become pregnant. **(M-S)**

In a patient who has had a stroke, the most serious complication is increasing intracranial pressure. **(M-S)**

If needed, cervical suturing is usually done between 14 and 18 weeks' gestation to reinforce an incompetent cervix and maintain pregnancy. The suturing is typically removed by 35 weeks' gestation. **(MAT)**

A patient with an intracranial hemorrhage should undergo arteriography to identify the site of the bleeding. **(M-S)**

Factors that affect the action of drugs include absorption, distribution, metabolism, and excretion. **(M-S)**

During the first trimester, a pregnant woman should avoid all drugs unless doing so would adversely affect her health. **(MAT)**

Before prescribing a drug for a woman of childbearing age, the prescriber should ask for the date of her last menstrual period and ask if she may be pregnant. **(M-S)**

Most drugs that a breast-feeding mother takes appear in breast milk. **(MAT)**

Acidosis may cause insulin resistance. **(M-S)**

A patient with glucose-6-phosphate dehydrogenase deficiency may have acute hemolytic anemia when given a sulfonamide. **(M-S)**

The Food and Drug Administration has established the following five categories of drugs based on their potential for causing birth defects: A, no evidence of risk; B, no risk found in animals, but no studies have been done in women; C, animal studies have shown an adverse effect, but the drug may be beneficial to women despite the potential risk; D, evidence of risk, but its benefits may outweigh its risks; and X, fetal anomalies noted, and the risks clearly outweigh the potential benefits.   (MAT)

The five basic activities of the digestive system are ingestion, movement of food, digestion, absorption, and defecation.   (M-S)

The nurse should use the bell of the stethoscope to listen for venous hums and cardiac murmurs.   (FND)

Signs and symptoms of acute pancreatitis include epigastric pain, vomiting, bluish discoloration of the left flank (Grey Turner's sign), bluish discoloration of the periumbilical area (Cullen's sign), low-grade fever, tachycardia, and hypotension.   (M-S)

A patient with a gastric ulcer may have gnawing or burning epigastric pain.   (M-S)

The nurse can assess a patient's general knowledge by asking questions such as "Who is the president of the United States?"   (FND)

To test the first cranial nerve (olfactory nerve), the nurse should ask the patient to close his eyes, occlude one nostril, and identify a nonirritating substance (such as peppermint or cinnamon) by smell. Then the nurse should repeat the test with the patient's other nostril occluded.   (M-S)

Salk and Sabin introduced the oral polio vaccine.   (M-S)

A patient with a disease of the cerebellum or posterior column has an ataxic gait that's characterized by staggering and inability to remain steady when standing with the feet together.   (M-S)

In trauma patients, improved outcome is directly related to early resuscitation, aggressive management of shock, and appropriate definitive care.   (M-S)

To check for leakage of cerebrospinal fluid, the nurse should inspect the patient's nose and ears. If the patient can sit up, the nurse should observe him for leakage as the patient leans forward.   (M-S)

For a child who is suspected of having Reye's syndrome, the nurse should ask the parents if the child received aspirin during the current or a recent illness.   (PED)

Locked-in syndrome is complete paralysis as a result of brain stem damage. Only the eyes can be moved voluntarily.   (M-S)

Neck dissection, or surgical removal of the cervical lymph nodes, is performed to prevent the spread of malignant tumors of the head and neck.
(M-S)

A patient with cholecystitis typically has right epigastric pain that may radiate to the right scapula or shoulder; nausea; and vomiting, especially after eating a heavy meal.   (M-S)

A patient with a ruptured ectopic pregnancy commonly has sharp pain in the lower abdomen, with spotting and cramping. She may have abdominal rigidity; rapid, shallow respirations; tachycardia; and shock.
(MAT)

Atropine is used preoperatively to reduce secretions.   (M-S)

Serum calcium levels are normally 4.5 to 5.5 mEq/L.   (M-S)

Suppressor T cells regulate overall immune response.   (M-S)

Serum levels of aspartate aminotransferase and alanine aminotransferase show whether the liver is adequately detoxifying drugs.   (M-S)

Serum sodium levels are normally 135 to 145 mEq/L.   (M-S)

Serum potassium levels are normally 3.5 to 5.0 mEq/L.   (M-S)

A patient who is taking prednisone (Deltasone) should consume a salt-restricted diet that's rich in potassium and protein.   (M-S)

When performing continuous ambulatory peritoneal dialysis, the nurse must use sterile technique when handling the catheter, send a peritoneal fluid sample for culture and sensitivity testing every 24 hours, and report signs of infection and fluid imbalance.   (M-S)

The Minnesota Multiphasic Personality Inventory consists of 550 statements for the subject to interpret. It assesses personality and detects disorders, such as depression and schizophrenia, in adolescents and adults.
(PSY)

▨ TORCH infections include toxoplasmosis, other diseases (chlamydia, group B beta-hemolytic streptococcus, syphilis, and varicella zoster), rubella, cytomegalovirus, and herpesvirus. Because these infections can harm an embryo or a fetus, the nurse must be alert for them when assessing a patient who is pregnant or considering pregnancy.   **(MAT)**

▨ An infant who is infected with human immunodeficiency virus during gestation typically begins to show signs and symptoms, such as fever, adenopathy, rash, diarrhea, and failure to thrive, between ages 2 and 4 months.   **(PED)**

▨ When working with patients who have acquired immunodeficiency syndrome, the nurse should wear goggles and a mask only if blood or another body fluid could splash onto the nurse's face.   **(M-S)**

▨ Blood spills that are infected with human immunodeficiency virus should be cleaned up with a 1:10 solution of sodium hypochlorite 5.25% (household bleach).   **(M-S)**

▨ *Raynaud's phenomenon* is intermittent ischemic attacks in the fingers or toes. It causes severe pallor and sometimes paresthesia and pain.   **(M-S)**

▨ Intussusception (prolapse of one bowel segment into the lumen of another) causes sudden epigastric pain, sausage-shaped abdominal swelling, passage of mucus and blood through the rectum, shock, and hypotension.   **(M-S)**

▨ The mechanics of delivery are engagement, descent and flexion, internal rotation, extension, external rotation, restitution, and expulsion.   **(MAT)**

▨ Bence Jones protein occurs almost exclusively in the urine of patients who have multiple myeloma.   **(M-S)**

▨ *Gaucher's disease* is an autosomal disorder that's characterized by abnormal accumulation of glucocerebrosides (lipid substances that contain glucose) in monocytes and macrocytes. It has three forms: Type 1 is the adult form, type 2 is the infantile form, and type 3 is the juvenile form.   **(M-S)**

▨ A patient with colon obstruction may have lower abdominal pain, constipation, increasing distention, and vomiting.   **(M-S)**

Cold packs are applied for the first 20 to 48 hours after an injury; then heat is applied. During cold application, the pack is applied for 20 minutes and then removed for 10 to 15 minutes to prevent reflex dilation (rebound phenomenon) and frostbite injury. **(FND)**

Colchicine (Colsalide) relieves inflammation and is used to treat gout. **(M-S)**

Some people have gout as a result of hyperuricemia because they can't metabolize and excrete purines normally. **(M-S)**

A normal sperm count is 20 to 150 million/ml. **(M-S)**

Organic brain syndrome is the most common form of mental illness in elderly patients. **(PSY)**

Clues to physical abuse of a child include inconsistent stories from parents about how the injuries occurred, lack of permission for the child to speak, wounds that don't match the stated cause of injury or multiple wounds at various stages of healing, and unexplained injuries. **(PED)**

A first-degree burn involves the stratum corneum layer of the epidermis and causes pain and redness. **(M-S)**

Sheehan's syndrome is hypopituitarism caused by a pituitary infarct after postpartum shock and hemorrhage. **(M-S)**

When caring for a patient who has had an asthma attack, the nurse should place the patient in Fowler's or semi-Fowler's position. **(M-S)**

In elderly patients, the incidence of noncompliance with prescribed drug therapy is high. Many elderly patients have diminished visual acuity, hearing loss, or forgetfulness, or need to take multiple drugs. **(M-S)**

Tuberculosis is a reportable communicable disease that's caused by infection with *Mycobacterium tuberculosis* (an acid-fast bacillus). **(M-S)**

For right-sided cardiac catheterization, the physician passes a multilumen catheter through the superior or inferior vena cava. **(M-S)**

A probable sign of pregnancy, McDonald's sign is characterized by an ease in flexing the body of the uterus against the cervix. **(MAT)**

Amenorrhea is a probable sign of pregnancy. **(MAT)**

A pregnant woman's partner should avoid introducing air into the vagina during oral sex because of the possibility of air embolism. (MAT)

The presence of human chorionic gonadotropin in the blood or urine is a probable sign of pregnancy. (MAT)

Radiography isn't usually used in a pregnant woman because it may harm the developing fetus. If radiography is essential, it should be performed only after 36 weeks' gestation. (MAT)

After a fracture, bone healing occurs in these stages: hematoma formation, cellular proliferation and callus formation, and ossification and remodeling. (M-S)

A pregnant patient who has had rupture of the membranes or who is experiencing vaginal bleeding shouldn't engage in sexual intercourse. (MAT)

A patient who is scheduled for positron emission tomography should avoid alcohol, tobacco, and caffeine for 24 hours before the test. (M-S)

Milia may occur as pinpoint spots over a neonate's nose. (MAT)

In a stroke, decreased oxygen destroys brain cells. (M-S)

The duration of a contraction is timed from the moment that the uterine muscle begins to tense to the moment that it reaches full relaxation. It's measured in seconds. (MAT)

A person who has an IQ of less than 20 is profoundly retarded and is considered a total-care patient. (PSY)

The union of a male and a female gamete produces a zygote, which divides into the fertilized ovum. (MAT)

A patient with glaucoma shouldn't receive atropine sulfate because it increases intraocular pressure. (M-S)

The nurse should instruct a patient who is hyperventilating to breathe into a paper bag. (M-S)

The first menstrual flow is called menarche and may be anovulatory (infertile). (MAT)

The pons is located above the medulla and consists of white matter (sensory and motor tracts) and gray matter (reflex centers). (FND)

▦ During intermittent positive-pressure breathing, the patient should bite down on the mouthpiece, breathe normally, and let the machine do the work. After inspiration, the patient should hold his breath for 3 or 4 seconds and exhale completely through the mouthpiece.   **(M-S)**

▦ The autonomic nervous system controls the smooth muscles.   **(FND)**

▦ Flexion contractures of the hips may occur in a patient who sits in a wheelchair for a long time.   **(M-S)**

▦ *Nystagmus* is rapid horizontal or rotating eye movement.   **(M-S)**

▦ After myelography, the patient should remain recumbent for 24 hours.   **(M-S)**

▦ The treatment of sprains and strains consists of applying ice immediately and elevating the arm or leg above heart level.   **(M-S)**

▦ An anticholinesterase agent shouldn't be prescribed for a patient who is taking morphine because it can potentiate the effect of morphine and cause respiratory depression.   **(M-S)**

▦ The primary purpose of play therapy for a hospitalized child is to allow him to express his feelings and frustrations.   **(PED)**

▦ *Reframing* is a therapeutic technique that's used to help depressed patients to view a situation in alternative ways.   **(PSY)**

▦ A correctly written patient goal expresses the desired patient behavior, criteria for measurement, time frame for achievement, and conditions under which the behavior will occur. It's developed in collaboration with the patient.   **(FND)**

▦ Percussion causes five basic notes: tympany (loud intensity, as heard over a gastric air bubble or puffed out cheek), hyperresonance (very loud, as heard over an emphysematous lung), resonance (loud, as heard over a normal lung), dullness (medium intensity, as heard over the liver or other solid organ), and flatness (soft, as heard over the thigh).   **(FND)**

▦ *Myopia* is nearsightedness. *Hyperopia* and *presbyopia* are two types of farsightedness.   **(M-S)**

▦ The optic disk is yellowish pink and circular, with a distinct border.   **(FND)**

The most effective contraceptive method is one that the woman selects for herself and uses consistently.   (M-S)

To perform Weber's test for bone conduction, a vibrating tuning fork is placed on top of the patient's head at midline. The patient should perceive the sound equally in both ears. In a patient who has conductive hearing loss, the sound is heard in (lateralizes to) the ear that has conductive loss.   (M-S)

In the Rinne test, bone conduction is tested by placing a vibrating tuning fork on the mastoid process of the temporal bone and air conduction is tested by holding the vibrating tuning fork $1/2''$ (1.3 cm) from the external auditory meatus. These tests are alternated, at different frequencies, until the tuning fork is no longer heard at one position.   (M-S)

A primary disability is caused by a pathologic process. A secondary disability is caused by inactivity.   (FND)

After an amputation, the stump may shrink because of muscle atrophy and decreased subcutaneous fat.   (M-S)

A patient who has deep vein thrombosis is given heparin for 7 to 10 days, followed by 12 weeks of warfarin (Coumadin) therapy.   (M-S)

After pneumonectomy, the patient should be positioned on the operative side or on his back, with his head slightly elevated.   (M-S)

To reduce the possibility of formation of new emboli or expansion of existing emboli, a patient with deep vein thrombosis should receive heparin.   (M-S)

Atherosclerosis is the most common cause of coronary artery disease. It usually involves the aorta and the femoral, coronary, and cerebral arteries.   (M-S)

Pulmonary embolism is a potentially fatal complication of deep vein thrombosis.   (M-S)

Chest pain is the most common symptom of pulmonary embolism.   (M-S)

The nurse should inform a patient who is taking phenazopyridine (Pyridium) that this drug colors urine orange or red.   (M-S)

■ Pneumothorax is a serious complication of central venous line placement; it's caused by inadvertent lung puncture.   (M-S)

■ *Pneumocystis carinii* pneumonia isn't considered contagious because it only affects patients who have a suppressed immune system.   (M-S)

■ To enhance drug absorption, the patient should take regular erythromycin tablets with a full glass of water 1 hour before or 2 hours after a meal or should take enteric-coated tablets with food. The patient should avoid taking either type of tablet with fruit juice.   (M-S)

■ Trismus, a sign of tetanus (lockjaw), causes painful spasms of the masticatory muscles, difficulty opening the mouth, neck rigidity and stiffness, and dysphagia.   (M-S)

■ Nurses are commonly held liable for failing to keep an accurate count of sponges and other devices during surgery.   (FND)

■ The best dietary sources of vitamin B_6 are liver, kidney, pork, soybeans, corn, and whole-grain cereals.   (FND)

■ The nurse should place the patient in an upright position for thoracentesis. If this isn't possible, the nurse should position the patient on the unaffected side.   (M-S)

■ If gravity flow is used, the nurse should hang a blood bag 3' (1 m) above the level of the planned venipuncture site.   (M-S)

■ The nurse should place a patient who has a closed chest drainage system in the semi-Fowler position.   (M-S)

■ Iron-rich foods, such as organ meats, nuts, legumes, dried fruit, green leafy vegetables, eggs, and whole grains, commonly have a low water content.   (FND)

■ If blood isn't transfused within 30 minutes, the nurse should return it to the blood bank because the refrigeration facilities on a nursing unit are inadequate for storing blood products.   (M-S)

■ Blood that's discolored and contains gas bubbles is contaminated with bacteria and shouldn't be transfused. Fifty percent of patients who receive contaminated blood die.   (M-S)

■ For massive, rapid blood transfusions and for exchange transfusions in neonates, blood should be warmed to 98.7° F (37° C).   (M-S)

▓ A *chest tube* permits air and fluid to drain from the pleural space. (M-S)

▓ A handheld resuscitation bag is an inflatable device that can be attached to a face mask or an endotracheal or tracheostomy tube. It allows manual delivery of oxygen to the lungs of a patient who can't breathe independently.   (M-S)

▓ Mechanical ventilation artificially controls or assists respiration. (M-S)

▓ The nurse should encourage a patient who has a closed chest drainage system to cough frequently and breathe deeply to help drain the pleural space and expand the lungs.   (M-S)

▓ Tracheal suction removes secretions from the trachea and bronchi with a suction catheter.   (M-S)

▓ During colostomy irrigation, the irrigation bag should be hung 18″ (45.7 cm) above the stoma.   (M-S)

▓ The water used for colostomy irrigation should be 100° to 105° F (37.8° to 40.6° C).   (M-S)

▓ An arterial embolism may cause pain, loss of sensory nerves, pallor, coolness, paralysis, pulselessness, or paresthesia in the affected arm or leg.
                                                                  (M-S)

▓ Respiratory alkalosis results from conditions that cause hyperventilation and reduce the carbon dioxide level in the arterial blood.   (M-S)

▓ Mineral oil is contraindicated in a patient with appendicitis, acute surgical abdomen, fecal impaction, or intestinal obstruction.   (M-S)

▓ When using a Y-type administration set to transfuse packed red blood cells (RBCs), the nurse can add normal saline solution to the bag to dilute the RBCs and make them less viscous.   (M-S)

▓ *Autotransfusion* is collection, filtration, and reinfusion of the patient's own blood.   (M-S)

▓ *Collaboration* is joint communication and decision making between nurses and physicians. It's designed to meet patients' needs by integrating the care regimens of both professions into one comprehensive approach.
                                                                  (FND)

▓ *Bradycardia* is a heart rate of fewer than 60 beats/minute.   (FND)

A *nursing diagnosis* is a statement of a patient's actual or potential health problem that can be resolved, diminished, or otherwise changed by nursing interventions. **(FND)**

During the assessment phase of the nursing process, the nurse collects and analyzes three types of data: health history, physical examination, and laboratory and diagnostic test data. **(FND)**

The patient's health history consists primarily of subjective data, information that's supplied by the patient. **(FND)**

The physical examination includes objective data obtained by inspection, palpation, percussion, and auscultation. **(FND)**

When documenting patient care, the nurse should write legibly, use only standard abbreviations, and sign each entry. The nurse should never destroy or attempt to obliterate documentation or leave vacant lines. **(FND)**

Factors that affect body temperature include time of day, age, physical activity, phase of menstrual cycle, and pregnancy. **(FND)**

The most accessible and commonly used artery for measuring a patient's pulse rate is the radial artery. To take the pulse rate, the artery is compressed against the radius. **(FND)**

In a resting adult, the normal pulse rate is 60 to 100 beats/minute. The rate is slightly faster in women than in men and much faster in children than in adults. **(FND)**

Prepared I.V. solutions fall into three general categories: isotonic, hypotonic, and hypertonic. Isotonic solutions have a solute concentration that's similar to body fluids; adding them to plasma doesn't change its osmolarity. Hypotonic solutions have a lower osmotic pressure than body fluids; adding them to plasma decreases its osmolarity. Hypertonic solutions have a higher osmotic pressure than body fluids; adding them to plasma increases its osmolarity. **(M-S)**

Stress incontinence is involuntary leakage of urine triggered by a sudden physical strain, such as a cough, sneeze, or quick movement. **(M-S)**

Laboratory test results are an objective form of assessment data. **(FND)**

Decreased renal function makes an elderly patient more susceptible to the development of renal calculi. **(M-S)**

The nurse should consider using shorter needles to inject drugs in elderly patients because these patients experience subcutaneous tissue redistribution and loss in areas, such as the buttocks and deltoid muscles. (M-S)

Urge incontinence is the inability to suppress a sudden urge to urinate. (M-S)

Total incontinence is continuous, uncontrollable leakage of urine as a result of the bladder's inability to retain urine. (M-S)

Protein, vitamin, and mineral needs usually remain constant as a person ages, but caloric requirements decrease. (M-S)

Four valves keep blood flowing in one direction in the heart: two atrioventricular valves (tricuspid and mitral) and two semilunar valves (pulmonic and aortic). (M-S)

An elderly patient's height may decrease because of narrowing of the intervertebral spaces and exaggerated spinal curvature. (M-S)

The measurement systems most commonly used in clinical practice are the metric system, apothecaries' system, and household system. (FND)

Before signing an informed consent form, the patient should know whether other treatment options are available and should understand what will occur during the preoperative, intraoperative, and postoperative phases; the risks involved; and the possible complications. The patient should also have a general idea of the time required from surgery to recovery. In addition, he should have an opportunity to ask questions. (FND)

A patient must sign a separate informed consent form for each procedure. (FND)

Constipation most commonly occurs when the urge to defecate is suppressed and the muscles associated with bowel movements remain contracted. (M-S)

Gout develops in four stages: asymptomatic, acute, intercritical, and chronic. (M-S)

▓ During percussion, the nurse uses quick, sharp tapping of the fingers or hands against body surfaces to produce sounds. This procedure is done to determine the size, shape, position, and density of underlying organs and tissues; elicit tenderness; or assess reflexes.   **(FND)**

▓ *Ballottement* is a form of light palpation involving gentle, repetitive bouncing of tissues against the hand and feeling their rebound.   **(FND)**

▓ A foot cradle keeps bed linen off the patient's feet to prevent skin irritation and breakdown, especially in a patient who has peripheral vascular disease or neuropathy.   **(FND)**

▓ *Gastric lavage* is flushing of the stomach and removal of ingested substances through a nasogastric tube. It's used to treat poisoning or drug overdose.   **(FND)**

▓ Common postoperative complications include hemorrhage, infection, hypovolemia, septicemia, septic shock, atelectasis, pneumonia, thrombophlebitis, and pulmonary embolism.   **(M-S)**

▓ An insulin pump delivers a continuous infusion of insulin into a selected subcutaneous site, commonly in the abdomen.   **(M-S)**

▓ During the evaluation step of the nursing process, the nurse assesses the patient's response to therapy.   **(FND)**

▓ A common symptom of salicylate (aspirin) toxicity is tinnitus (ringing in the ears).   **(M-S)**

▓ A frostbitten extremity must be thawed rapidly, even if definitive treatment must be delayed.   **(M-S)**

▓ Bruits commonly indicate life- or limb-threatening vascular disease.
(FND)

▓ A patient with Raynaud's disease shouldn't smoke cigarettes or other tobacco products.   **(M-S)**

▓ *O.U.* means each eye. *O.D.* is the right eye, and *O.S.* is the left eye.
(FND)

▓ Raynaud's disease is a primary arteriospastic disorder that has no known cause. Raynaud's phenomenon, however, is caused by another disorder such as scleroderma.   **(M-S)**

■ To remove a foreign body from the eye, the nurse should irrigate the eye with sterile normal saline solution.   **(M-S)**

■ When irrigating the eye, the nurse should direct the solution toward the lower conjunctival sac.   **(M-S)**

■ Emergency care for a corneal injury caused by a caustic substance is flushing the eye with copious amounts of water for 20 to 30 minutes. **(M-S)**

■ To remove a patient's artificial eye, the nurse depresses the lower lid.
                                                                                  (FND)

■ The nurse should use a warm saline solution to clean an artificial eye.
                                                                                  (FND)

■ *Debridement* is mechanical, chemical, or surgical removal of necrotic tissue from a wound.   **(M-S)**

■ Severe pain after cataract surgery indicates bleeding in the eye.   **(M-S)**

■ A bivalve cast is cut into anterior and posterior portions to allow skin inspection.   **(M-S)**

■ After ear irrigation, the nurse should place the patient on the affected side to permit gravity to drain fluid that remains in the ear.   **(M-S)**

■ In evaluating dehydration in an infant, the nurse should assess skin turgor on the inner thigh.   **(PED)**

■ A thready pulse is very fine and scarcely perceptible.   **(FND)**

■ If a patient with an indwelling catheter has abdominal discomfort, the nurse should assess for bladder distention, which may be caused by catheter blockage.   **(M-S)**

■ Continuous bladder irrigation helps prevent urinary tract obstruction by flushing out small blood clots that form after prostate or bladder surgery.
                                                                                  (M-S)

■ The nurse should remove an indwelling catheter when bladder decompression is no longer needed, when the catheter is obstructed, or when the patient can resume voiding. The longer a catheter remains in place, the greater the risk of urinary tract infection.   **(M-S)**

In an adult, the extent of a burn injury is determined by using the Rule of Nines: the head and neck are counted as 9%; each arm, as 9%; each leg, as 18%; the back of the trunk, as 18%; the front of the trunk, as 18%; and the perineum, as 1%. **(M-S)**

A deep partial-thickness burn affects the epidermis and dermis.   **(M-S)**

Axillary temperature is usually 1° F lower than oral temperature. **(FND)**

After suctioning a tracheostomy tube, the nurse must document the color, amount, consistency, and odor of secretions.   **(FND)**

In a patient who is having an asthma attack, nursing interventions include administering oxygen and bronchodilators as prescribed, placing the patient in the semi-Fowler position, encouraging diaphragmatic breathing, and helping the patient to relax.   **(M-S)**

On a drug prescription, the abbreviation p.c. means that the drug should be administered after meals.   **(FND)**

After bladder irrigation, the nurse should document the amount, color, and clarity of the urine and the presence of clots or sediment.   **(FND)**

Prostate cancer is usually fatal if bone metastasis occurs.   **(M-S)**

Laws regarding patient self-determination vary from state to state. Therefore, the nurse must be familiar with the laws of the state in which she works.   **(FND)**

Gauge is the inside diameter of a needle: the smaller the gauge, the larger the diameter.   **(FND)**

An adult normally has 32 permanent teeth.   **(FND)**

After turning a patient, the nurse should document the position used, the time that the patient was turned, and the findings of skin assessment.   **(FND)**

A strict vegetarian needs vitamin B_{12} supplements because animals and animal products are the only source of this vitamin.   **(M-S)**

PERRLA is an abbreviation for normal pupil assessment findings: pupils equal, round, and reactive to light with accommodation.   **(FND)**

When percussing a patient's chest for postural drainage, the nurse's hands should be cupped.   **(FND)**

■ Regular insulin is the only type of insulin that can be mixed with other types of insulin and can be given I.V. **(M-S)**

■ If a patient pulls out the outer tracheostomy tube, the nurse should hold the tracheostomy open with a surgical dilator until the physician provides appropriate care. **(M-S)**

■ When measuring a patient's pulse, the nurse should assess its rate, rhythm, quality, and strength. **(FND)**

■ Before transferring a patient from a bed to a wheelchair, the nurse should push the wheelchair's footrests to the sides and lock its wheels. **(FND)**

■ When assessing respirations, the nurse should document their rate, rhythm, depth, and quality. **(FND)**

■ For a subcutaneous injection, the nurse should use a ⁵/₈" 25G needle. **(FND)**

■ The *medulla oblongata* is the part of the brain that controls the respiratory center. **(M-S)**

■ For an unconscious patient, the nurse should perform passive range-of-motion exercises every 2 to 4 hours. **(M-S)**

■ A timed-release drug isn't recommended for use in a patient who has an ileostomy because it releases the drug at different rates along the GI tract. **(M-S)**

■ The notation "AA & O × 3" indicates that the patient is awake, alert, and oriented to person (knows who he is), place (knows where he is), and time (knows the date and time). **(FND)**

■ *Fluid intake* includes all fluids taken by mouth, including foods that are liquid at room temperature, such as gelatin, custard, and ice cream; I.V. fluids; and fluids administered in feeding tubes. Fluid output includes urine, vomitus, and drainage (such as from a nasogastric tube or from a wound) as well as blood loss, diarrhea or feces, and perspiration. **(FND)**

■ The nurse isn't required to wear gloves when applying nitroglycerin paste; however, she should wash her hands after applying this drug. **(M-S)**

■ Before excretory urography, a patient's fluid intake is usually restricted after midnight. **(M-S)**

After administering an intradermal injection, the nurse shouldn't massage the area because massage can irritate the site and interfere with results.
(FND)

When administering an intradermal injection, the nurse should hold the syringe almost flat against the patient's skin (at about a 15-degree angle), with the bevel up.
(FND)

To obtain an accurate blood pressure, the nurse should inflate the manometer to 20 to 30 mm Hg above the disappearance of the radial pulse before releasing the cuff pressure.
(FND)

A sodium polystyrene sulfonate (Kayexalate) enema, which exchanges sodium ions for potassium ions, is used to decrease the potassium level in a patient who has hyperkalemia.
(M-S)

If the color of a stoma is much lighter than when previously assessed, decreased circulation to the stoma should be suspected.
(M-S)

Massage is contraindicated in a leg with a blood clot because it may dislodge the clot.
(M-S)

The first place a nurse can detect jaundice in an adult is in the sclera.
(M-S)

Jaundice is caused by excessive levels of conjugated or unconjugated bilirubin in the blood.
(M-S)

Mydriatic drugs are used primarily to dilate the pupils for intraocular examinations.
(M-S)

After eye surgery, the patient should be placed on the unaffected side.
(M-S)

When assigning tasks to a licensed practical nurse, the registered nurse should delegate tasks that are considered bedside nursing care, such as taking vital signs, changing simple dressings, and giving baths.
(M-S)

Deep calf pain on dorsiflexion of the foot is a positive Homans' sign, which suggests venous thrombosis or thrombophlebitis.
(M-S)

Ultra-short-acting barbiturates, such as thiopental (Pentothal), are used as injection anesthetics when a short duration of anesthesia is needed such as outpatient surgery.
(M-S)

Atropine sulfate may be used as a preanesthetic drug to reduce secretions and minimize vagal reflexes. **(M-S)**

For a patient with infectious mononucleosis, the nursing care plan should emphasize strict bed rest during the acute febrile stage to ensure adequate rest. **(M-S)**

During the acute phase of infectious mononucleosis, the patient should curtail activities to minimize the possibility of rupturing the enlarged spleen. **(M-S)**

Daily application of a long-acting, transdermal nitroglycerin patch is a convenient, effective way to prevent chronic angina. **(M-S)**

Fluoxetine (Prozac), sertraline (Zoloft), and paroxetine (Paxil) are serotonin reuptake inhibitors used to treat depression. **(PSY)**

The nurse must wear a cap, gloves, a gown, and a mask when providing wound care to a patient with third-degree burns. **(M-S)**

The nurse should expect to administer an analgesic before bathing a burn patient. **(M-S)**

The passage of black, tarry feces (melena) is a common sign of lower GI bleeding, but also may occur in patients who have upper GI bleeding. **(M-S)**

The nurse should count an irregular pulse for 1 full minute. **(FND)**

Spermatozoa (or their fragments) remain in the vagina for 72 hours after sexual intercourse. **(MAT)**

A patient who has a gastric ulcer should avoid taking aspirin and aspirin-containing products because they can irritate the gastric mucosa. **(M-S)**

A patient who is vomiting while lying down should be placed in a lateral position to prevent aspiration of vomitus. **(FND)**

While administering chemotherapy agents with an I.V. line, the nurse should discontinue the infusion at the first sign of extravasation. **(M-S)**

A low-fiber diet may contribute to the development of hemorrhoids. **(M-S)**

▓ A patient who has abdominal pain shouldn't receive an analgesic until the cause of the pain is determined. **(M-S)**

▓ If surgery requires hair removal, the recommendation of the Centers for Disease Control and Prevention is that a depilatory be used to avoid skin abrasions and cuts. **(M-S)**

▓ For nasotracheal suctioning, the nurse should set wall suction at 50 to 95 mm Hg for an infant, 95 to 115 mm Hg for a child, or 80 to 120 mm Hg for an adult. **(M-S)**

▓ The hallmark of tetralogy of Fallot is cyanosis, which usually appears several months after birth, but may be present at birth if the neonate has severe pulmonary stenosis. **(PED)**

▓ After a myocardial infarction, a change in pulse rate and rhythm may signal the onset of fatal arrhythmias. **(M-S)**

▓ Treatment of epistaxis includes nasal packing, ice packs, cautery with silver nitrate, and pressure on the nares. **(M-S)**

▓ *Prophylaxis* is disease prevention. **(FND)**

▓ *Palliative treatment* relieves or reduces the intensity of uncomfortable symptoms, but doesn't cure the causative disorder. **(M-S)**

▓ Placing a postoperative patient in an upright position too quickly may cause hypotension. **(M-S)**

▓ *Body alignment* is achieved when body parts are in proper relation to their natural position. **(FND)**

▓ Verapamil (Calan) and diltiazem (Cardizem) slow the inflow of calcium to the heart, thereby decreasing the risk of supraventricular tachycardia. **(M-S)**

▓ Trust is the foundation of a nurse-patient relationship. **(FND)**

▓ *Blood pressure* is the force exerted by the circulating volume of blood on the arterial walls. **(FND)**

▓ After cardiopulmonary bypass graft, the patient will perform turning, coughing, deep breathing, and wound splinting, and will use assistive breathing devices. **(M-S)**

A patient who is exposed to hepatitis B should receive 0.06 ml/kg I.M. of immune globulin within 72 hours after exposure and a repeat dose at 28 days after exposure. **(M-S)**

The nurse should advise a patient who is undergoing radiation therapy not to remove the markings on the skin made by the radiation therapist because they are landmarks for treatment. **(M-S)**

The most common symptom of osteoarthritis is joint pain that's relieved by rest, especially if the pain occurs after exercise or weight bearing. **(M-S)**

Malpractice is a professional's wrongful conduct, improper discharge of duties, or failure to meet standards of care that causes harm to another. **(FND)**

In adults, urine volume normally ranges from 800 to 2,000 ml/day and averages between 1,200 and 1,500 ml/day. **(M-S)**

As a general rule, nurses can't refuse a patient care assignment; however, in most states, they may refuse to participate in abortions. **(FND)**

A nurse can be found negligent if a patient is injured because the nurse failed to perform a duty that a reasonable and prudent person would perform or because the nurse performed an act that a reasonable and prudent person wouldn't perform. **(FND)**

Directly applied moist heat softens crusts and exudates, penetrates deeper than dry heat, doesn't dry the skin, and is usually more comfortable for the patient. **(M-S)**

Tetracyclines are seldom considered drugs of choice for most common bacterial infections because their overuse has led to the emergence of tetracycline-resistant bacteria. **(M-S)**

Because light degrades nitroprusside (Nitropress), the drug must be shielded from light. For example, an I.V. bag that contains nitroprusside sodium should be wrapped in foil. **(M-S)**

Cephalosporins should be used cautiously in patients who are allergic to penicillin. These patients are more susceptible to hypersensitivity reactions. **(M-S)**

■ If chloramphenicol and penicillin must be administered concomitantly, the nurse should give the penicillin 1 or more hours before the chloramphenicol to avoid a reduction in penicillin's bactericidal activity.

(M-S)

■ The erythrocyte sedimentation rate measures the distance and speed at which erythrocytes in whole blood fall in a vertical tube in 1 hour. The rate at which they fall to the bottom of the tube corresponds to the degree of inflammation. (M-S)

■ When teaching a patient with myasthenia gravis about pyridostigmine (Mestinon) therapy, the nurse should stress the importance of taking the drug exactly as prescribed, on time, and in evenly spaced doses to prevent a relapse and maximize the effect of the drug. (M-S)

■ If an antibiotic must be administered into a peripheral heparin lock, the nurse should flush the site with normal saline solution after the infusion to maintain I.V. patency. (M-S)

■ The nurse should instruct a patient with angina to take a nitroglycerin tablet before anticipated stress or exercise or, if the angina is nocturnal, at bedtime. (M-S)

■ Arterial blood gas analysis evaluates gas exchange in the lungs (alveolar ventilation) by measuring the partial pressures of oxygen and carbon dioxide and the pH of an arterial sample. (M-S)

■ The normal serum magnesium level ranges from 1.5 to 2.5 mEq/L.

(M-S)

■ Patient preparation for a total cholesterol test includes an overnight fast and abstinence from alcohol for 24 hours before the test. (M-S)

■ The fasting plasma glucose test measures glucose levels after a 12- to 14-hour fast. (M-S)

■ Normal blood pH ranges from 7.35 to 7.45. A blood pH higher than 7.45 indicates alkalemia; one lower than 7.35 indicates acidemia. (M-S)

■ During an acid perfusion test, a small amount of weak hydrochloric acid solution is infused with a nasoesophageal tube. A positive test result (pain after infusion) suggests reflux esophagitis. (M-S)

■ Normally, the partial pressure of arterial carbon dioxide ($Paco_2$) ranges from 35 to 45 mm Hg. A $Paco_2$ greater than 45 mm Hg indicates acidemia as a result of hypoventilation; one less than 35 mm Hg indicates alkalemia as a result of hyperventilation. **(M-S)**

■ Red cell indices aid in the diagnosis and classification of anemia. **(M-S)**

■ Normally, the partial pressure of arterial oxygen (Pao_2) ranges from 80 to 100 mm Hg. A Pao_2 of 50 to 80 mm Hg indicates respiratory insufficiency. A Pao_2 of less than 50 mm Hg indicates respiratory failure.
(M-S)

■ The white blood cell (WBC) differential evaluates WBC distribution and morphology and provides more specific information about a patient's immune system than the WBC count. **(M-S)**

■ An exercise stress test (treadmill test, exercise electrocardiogram) continues until the patient reaches a predetermined target heart rate or experiences chest pain, fatigue, or other signs of exercise intolerance. **(M-S)**

■ Alterable risk factors for coronary artery disease include cigarette smoking, hypertension, high cholesterol or triglyceride levels, and diabetes.
(M-S)

■ The *mediastinum* is the space between the lungs that contains the heart, esophagus, trachea, and other structures. **(M-S)**

■ Major complications of acute myocardial infarction include arrhythmias, acute heart failure, cardiogenic shock, thromboembolism, and left ventricular rupture. **(M-S)**

■ The *sinoatrial node* is a cluster of hundreds of cells located in the right atrial wall, near the opening of the superior vena cava. **(M-S)**

■ For one-person cardiopulmonary resuscitation, the ratio of compressions to ventilations is 15:2. **(M-S)**

■ For two-person cardiopulmonary resuscitation, the ratio of compressions to ventilations is 5:1. **(M-S)**

■ A patient who has pulseless ventricular tachycardia is a candidate for cardioversion. **(M-S)**

- *Echocardiography*, a noninvasive test that directs ultra-high-frequency sound waves through the chest wall and into the heart, evaluates cardiac structure and function and can show valve deformities, tumors, septal defects, pericardial effusion, and hypertrophic cardiomyopathy. **(M-S)**

- *Ataxia* is impaired ability to coordinate movements. It's caused by a cerebellar or spinal cord lesion. **(M-S)**

- On an electrocardiogram strip, each small block on the horizontal axis represents 0.04 second. Each large block (composed of five small blocks) represents 0.2 second. **(M-S)**

- Starling's law states that the force of contraction of each heartbeat depends on the length of the muscle fibers of the heart wall. **(M-S)**

- The therapeutic blood level for digoxin is 0.5 to 2.5 ng/ml. **(M-S)**

- Pancrelipase (Pancrease) is used to treat cystic fibrosis and chronic pancreatitis. **(M-S)**

- Treatment for mild to moderate varicose veins includes antiembolism stockings and an exercise program that includes walking to minimize venous pooling. **(M-S)**

- According to Erikson, a young adult (ages 19 to 35) is in the developmental stage of intimacy versus isolation. **(PED)**

- States have enacted Good Samaritan laws to encourage professionals to provide medical assistance at the scene of an accident without fear of a lawsuit arising from the assistance. These laws don't apply to care provided in a health care facility. **(FND)**

- A physician should sign verbal and telephone orders within the time established by facility policy, usually 24 hours. **(FND)**

- A competent adult has the right to refuse lifesaving medical treatment; however, the individual should be fully informed of the consequences of his refusal. **(FND)**

- An intoxicated patient isn't considered competent to refuse required medical treatment and shouldn't be allowed to check out of a hospital against medical advice. **(M-S)**

- The primary difference between the pain of angina and that of a myocardial infarction is its duration. **(M-S)**

Although a patient's health record, or chart, is the health care facility's physical property, its contents belong to the patient.   **(FND)**

Before a patient's health record can be released to a third party, the patient or the patient's legal guardian must give written consent.   **(FND)**

Under the Controlled Substances Act, every dose of a controlled drug that's dispensed by the pharmacy must be accounted for, whether the dose was administered to a patient or discarded accidentally.   **(FND)**

A nurse can't perform duties that violate a rule or regulation established by a state licensing board, even if they are authorized by a health care facility or physician.   **(FND)**

To minimize interruptions during a patient interview, the nurse should select a private room, preferably one with a door that can be closed.
(FND)

In categorizing nursing diagnoses, the nurse addresses life-threatening problems first, followed by potentially life-threatening concerns.
(FND)

The major components of a nursing care plan are outcome criteria (patient goals) and nursing interventions.   **(FND)**

Standing orders, or *protocols*, establish guidelines for treating a specific disease or set of symptoms.   **(FND)**

Prolactin stimulates and sustains milk production.   **(MAT)**

Gynecomastia is excessive mammary gland development and increased breast size in boys and men.   **(M-S)**

The early stage of Alzheimer's disease lasts 2 to 4 years. Patients have inappropriate affect, transient paranoia, disorientation to time, memory loss, careless dressing, and impaired judgment.   **(PSY)**

The middle stage of Alzheimer's disease lasts 4 to 7 years and is marked by profound personality changes, loss of independence, disorientation, confusion, inability to recognize family members, and nocturnal restlessness.   **(PSY)**

The last stage of Alzheimer's disease occurs during the final year of life and is characterized by a blank facial expression, seizures, loss of appetite, emaciation, irritability, and total dependence.   **(PSY)**

- Classic symptoms of Graves' disease are an enlarged thyroid, nervousness, heat intolerance, weight loss despite increased appetite, sweating, diarrhea, tremor, and palpitations. **(M-S)**

- Generalized malaise is a common symptom of viral and bacterial infections and depressive disorders. **(M-S)**

- Vitamin C and protein are the most important nutrients for wound healing. **(M-S)**

- A patient who has portal hypertension should receive vitamin K to promote active thrombin formation by the liver. Thrombin reduces the risk of bleeding. **(M-S)**

- The nurse should administer a sedative cautiously to a patient with cirrhosis because the damaged liver can't metabolize drugs effectively. **(M-S)**

- Beta-hemolytic streptococcal infections should be treated aggressively to prevent glomerulonephritis, rheumatic fever, and other complications. **(M-S)**

- The most common nosocomial infection is a urinary tract infection. **(M-S)**

- The nurse should implement strict isolation precautions to protect a patient with a third-degree burn that's infected by *Staphylococcus aureus*. **(M-S)**

- A patient who is undergoing external radiation therapy shouldn't apply cream or lotion to the treatment site. **(M-S)**

- Strabismus is a normal finding in a neonate. **(MAT)**

- The most common vascular complication of diabetes mellitus is atherosclerosis. **(M-S)**

- Insulin deficiency may cause hyperglycemia. **(M-S)**

- Signs of Parkinson's disease include drooling, a masklike expression, and a propulsive gait. **(M-S)**

- I.V. cholangiography is contraindicated in a patient with hyperthyroidism, severe renal or hepatic damage, tuberculosis, or iodine hypersensitivity. **(M-S)**

In assessing a patient's heart, the nurse normally finds the point of maximal impulse at the fifth intercostal space, near the apex.   (FND)

The S_1 heard on auscultation is caused by closure of the mitral and tricuspid valves.   (FND)

Threatening a patient with an injection for failing to take an oral drug is an example of assault.   (PSY)

Mirrors should be removed from the room of a patient who has disfiguring wounds such as facial burns.   (M-S)

A patient who has gouty arthritis should increase fluid intake to prevent calculi formation.   (M-S)

Anxiety is the most common cause of chest pain.   (M-S)

A patient who is following a low-salt diet should avoid canned vegetables.   (M-S)

Bananas are a good source of potassium and should be included in a low-salt diet for patients who are taking a loop diuretic such as furosemide (Lasix).   (M-S)

The nurse should encourage a patient who is at risk for pneumonia to turn frequently, cough, and breathe deeply. These actions mobilize pulmonary secretions, promote alveolar gas exchange, and help prevent atelectasis.   (M-S)

The nurse should notify the physician whenever a patient's blood pressure reaches 180/100 mm Hg.   (M-S)

Buck's traction is used to immobilize and reduce spasms in a fractured hip.   (M-S)

For a patient with a fractured hip, the nurse should assess neurocirculatory status every 2 hours.   (M-S)

When caring for a patient with a fractured hip, the nurse should use pillows or a trochanter roll to maintain abduction.   (M-S)

Orthopnea is a symptom of left-sided heart failure.   (M-S)

Although a fiberglass cast is more durable and dries more quickly than a plaster cast, it typically causes skin irritation.   (M-S)

▨ In an immobilized patient, the major circulatory complication is pulmonary embolism.   (M-S)

▨ To relieve edema in a fractured limb, the patient should keep the limb elevated.   (M-S)

▨ I.V. antibiotics are the treatment of choice for a patient with osteomyelitis.   (M-S)

▨ A postpartum patient may resume sexual intercourse after the perineal or uterine wounds heal (usually within 4 weeks after delivery).   (MAT)

▨ Blue dye in cimetidine (Tagamet) can cause a false-positive result on a fecal occult blood test such as a Hemoccult test.   (M-S)

▨ A pregnant staff member shouldn't be assigned to work with a patient who has cytomegalovirus infection because the virus can be transmitted to the fetus.   (MAT)

▨ The nurse should suspect elder abuse if wounds are inconsistent with the patient's history, multiple wounds are present, or wounds are in different stages of healing.   (M-S)

▨ *Fetal demise* is death of the fetus after viability.   (MAT)

▨ Immediately after amputation, patient care includes monitoring drainage from the stump, positioning the affected limb, assisting with exercises prescribed by a physical therapist, and wrapping and conditioning the stump.   (M-S)

▨ Respiratory distress syndrome develops in premature neonates because their alveoli lack surfactant.   (MAT)

▨ A patient who is prone to constipation should increase his bulk intake by eating whole-grain cereals and fresh fruits and vegetables.   (M-S)

▨ The most common method of inducing labor after artificial rupture of the membranes is oxytocin (Pitocin) infusion.   (MAT)

▨ In the pelvic examination of a sexual assault victim, the speculum should be lubricated with water. Commercial lubricants retard sperm motility and interfere with specimen collection and analysis.   (M-S)

▨ For a terminally ill patient, physical comfort is the top priority in nursing care.   (M-S)

Dorsiflexion of the foot provides immediate relief of leg cramps. (M-S)

After cardiac surgery, the patient should limit daily sodium intake to 2 g and daily cholesterol intake to 300 mg.   (M-S)

After the amniotic membranes rupture, the initial nursing action is to assess the fetal heart rate.   (MAT)

Bleeding after intercourse is an early sign of cervical cancer.   (M-S)

Oral antidiabetic agents, such as chlorpropamide (Diabinese) and tolbutamide (Orinase), stimulate insulin release from beta cells in the islets of Langerhans of the pancreas.   (M-S)

When visiting a patient who has a radiation implant, family members and friends must limit their stay to 10 minutes. Visitors and nurses who are pregnant are restricted from entering the room.   (M-S)

Common causes of vaginal infection include using an antibiotic, an oral contraceptive, or a corticosteroid; wearing tight-fitting panty hose; and having sexual intercourse with an infected partner.   (M-S)

A patient with a radiation implant should remain in isolation until the implant is removed. To minimize radiation exposure, which increases with time, the nurse should carefully plan the time spent with the patient.   (M-S)

Among cultural groups, Native Americans have the lowest incidence of cancer.   (M-S)

The kidneys filter blood, selectively reabsorb substances that are needed to maintain the constancy of body fluid, and excrete metabolic wastes.   (M-S)

Reexamination of life goals is a major developmental task during middle adulthood.   (PSY)

To prevent straining during defecation, docusate (Colace) is the laxative of choice for patients who are recovering from a myocardial infarction, rectal or cardiac surgery, or postpartum constipation.   (M-S)

Acute alcohol withdrawal causes anorexia, insomnia, headache, and restlessness and escalates to a syndrome that's characterized by agitation, disorientation, vivid hallucinations, and tremors of the hands, feet, legs, and tongue.   (PSY)

In a hospitalized alcoholic, alcohol withdrawal delirium most commonly occurs 3 to 4 days after admission.   (PSY)

Confrontation is a communication technique in which the nurse points out discrepancies between the patient's words and his nonverbal behaviors.   (PSY)

Telangiectatic nevi (stork bites) are normal neonatal skin lesions that are characterized by flat red or purple areas on the back of the neck, upper eyelids, upper lip, and bridge of the nose. They regress by age 2.   (PED)

After prostate surgery, a patient's primary sources of pain are bladder spasms and irritation in the area around the catheter.   (M-S)

Toxoplasmosis is more likely to affect a pregnant cat owner than other pregnant women because cat feces in the litter box harbor the infecting organism.   (M-S)

The most common reasons for cesarean birth are malpresentation, fetal distress, cephalopelvic disproportion, pregnancy-induced hypertension, previous cesarean birth, and inadequate progress in labor.   (MAT)

Amniocentesis increases the risk of spontaneous abortion, trauma to the fetus or placenta, premature labor, infection, and Rh sensitization of the fetus.   (MAT)

After amniocentesis, abdominal cramping or spontaneous vaginal bleeding may indicate complications.   (MAT)

To prevent her from developing Rh antibodies, an Rh-negative primigravida should receive $Rh_o(D)$ immune globulin (RhoGAM) after delivering an Rh-positive neonate.   (MAT)

If a pregnant patient's test results are negative for glucose but positive for acetone, the nurse should assess the patient's diet for inadequate caloric intake.   (MAT)

Calcium deficiency and lack of proper exercise can cause leg cramps during pregnancy.   (MAT)

Good food sources of folic acid include green leafy vegetables, liver, and legumes.   (M-S)

Rubella infection in a pregnant patient, especially during the first trimester, can lead to spontaneous abortion or stillbirth as well as fetal cardiac and other birth defects. **(MAT)**

The *Glasgow Coma Scale* evaluates verbal, eye, and motor responses to determine the patient's level of consciousness. **(M-S)**

The nurse should place an unconscious patient in low Fowler's position for intermittent nasogastric tube feedings. **(M-S)**

Laënnec's (alcoholic) cirrhosis is the most common type of cirrhosis. **(M-S)**

In decorticate posturing, the patient's arms are adducted and flexed, with the wrists and fingers flexed on the chest. The legs are extended stiffly and rotated internally, with plantar flexion of the feet. **(M-S)**

For a patient with substance-induced delirium, the time of drug ingestion can help to determine whether the drug can be evacuated from the body. **(PSY)**

A pregnant patient should take an iron supplement to help prevent anemia. **(MAT)**

Direct antiglobulin (direct Coombs') test is used to detect maternal antibodies attached to red blood cells in the neonate. **(MAT)**

The most common intra-abdominal tumor in children is Wilms' tumor (nephroblastoma). **(PED)**

Candidates for surgery should receive nothing by mouth from midnight of the day before surgery unless cleared by a physician. **(M-S)**

Nausea and vomiting during the first trimester of pregnancy are caused by rising levels of the hormone human chorionic gonadotropin. **(MAT)**

In an infant, feeding problems, such as fatigue, tachypnea, and irritability during feeding, may be early signs of a congenital heart defect. **(PED)**

Meperidine (Demerol) is an effective analgesic to relieve the pain of nephrolithiasis (urinary calculi). **(M-S)**

An injured patient with thrombocytopenia is at risk for life-threatening internal and external hemorrhage. **(M-S)**

▧ The Trendelenburg test is used to check for unilateral hip dislocation. (M-S)

▧ As soon as possible after death, the patient should be placed in the supine position, with the arms at the sides and the head on a pillow.   (M-S)

▧ Vascular resistance depends on blood viscosity, vessel length and, most important, inside vessel diameter.   (M-S)

▧ A below-the-knee amputation leaves the knee intact for prosthesis application and allows a more normal gait than above-the-knee amputation. (M-S)

▧ Cerebrospinal fluid flows through and protects the four ventricles of the brain, the subarachnoid space, and the spinal canal.   (M-S)

▧ Sodium regulates extracellular osmolality.   (M-S)

▧ The heart and brain can maintain blood circulation in the early stages of shock.   (M-S)

▧ After limb amputation, narcotic analgesics may not relieve "phantom limb" pain.   (M-S)

▧ A patient who receives multiple blood transfusions is at risk for hypocalcemia.   (M-S)

▧ Syphilis initially causes painless chancres (small, fluid-filled lesions) on the genitals and sometimes on other parts of the body.   (M-S)

▧ Exposure to a radioactive source is controlled by time (limiting time spent with the patient), distance (from the patient), and shield (a lead apron). (M-S)

▧ Jaundice is a sign of dysfunction, not a disease.   (M-S)

▧ Severe jaundice can cause brain stem dysfunction if the unconjugated bilirubin level in blood is elevated to 20 to 25 mg/dl.   (M-S)

▧ The patient should take cimetidine (Tagamet) with meals to help ensure a consistent therapeutic effect.   (M-S)

▧ When caring for a patient with jaundice, the nurse should relieve pruritus by providing a soothing lotion or a baking soda bath and should prevent injury by keeping the patient's fingernails short.   (M-S)

■ Type B hepatitis, which is usually transmitted parenterally, also can be spread through contact with human secretions and feces. **(M-S)**

■ Insulin is a naturally occurring hormone that's secreted by the beta cells of the islets of Langerhans in the pancreas in response to a rise in the blood glucose level. **(M-S)**

■ Diabetes mellitus is a chronic endocrine disorder that's characterized by insulin deficiency or resistance to insulin by body tissues. **(M-S)**

■ A diagnosis of diabetes mellitus is based on the classic symptoms (polyuria, polyphagia, weight loss, and polydipsia) and a random blood glucose level of more than 200 mg/dl or a fasting plasma glucose level of more than 140 mg/dl when tested on two separate occasions. **(M-S)**

■ A patient with non–insulin-dependent (type 2) diabetes mellitus produces some insulin and normally doesn't need exogenous insulin supplementation. Most patients with this type of diabetes respond well to oral antidiabetic agents, which stimulate the pancreas to increase the synthesis and release of insulin. **(M-S)**

■ A patient with insulin-dependent (type 1) diabetes mellitus can't produce endogenous insulin and requires exogenous insulin administration to meet the body's needs. **(M-S)**

■ Rapid-acting insulins are clear; intermediate- and long-acting insulins are turbid (cloudy). **(M-S)**

■ Rapid-acting insulins begin to act in 30 to 60 minutes, reach a peak concentration in 2 to 10 hours, and have a duration of action of 5 to 16 hours. **(M-S)**

■ The best times to test a diabetic patient's glucose level are before each meal and at bedtime. **(M-S)**

■ Intermediate-acting insulins begin to act in 1 to 2 hours, reach a peak concentration in 4 to 15 hours, and have a duration of action of 22 to 28 hours. **(M-S)**

■ Long-acting insulins begin to act in 4 to 8 hours, reach a peak concentration in 10 to 30 hours, and have a duration of action of 36 hours or more. **(M-S)**

■ If the results of a nonfasting glucose test show above-normal glucose levels after glucose administration, but the patient has normal plasma glucose levels otherwise, the patient has impaired glucose tolerance. (M-S)

■ Insulin requirements are increased by growth, pregnancy, increased food intake, stress, surgery, infection, illness, increased insulin antibodies, and some drugs. (M-S)

■ Insulin requirements are decreased by hypothyroidism, decreased food intake, exercise, and some drugs. (M-S)

■ Hypoglycemia occurs when the blood glucose level is less than 50 mg/dl. (M-S)

■ An insulin-resistant patient is one who requires more than 200 units of insulin daily. (M-S)

■ Hypoglycemia may occur 1 to 3 hours after the administration of a rapid-acting insulin, 4 to 18 hours after the administration of an intermediate-acting insulin, and 18 to 30 hours after the administration of a long-acting insulin. (M-S)

■ When the blood glucose level decreases rapidly, the patient may experience sweating, tremors, pallor, tachycardia, and palpitations. (M-S)

■ Objective signs of hypoglycemia include slurred speech, lack of coordination, staggered gait, seizures, and possibly, coma. (M-S)

■ A conscious patient who has hypoglycemia should receive sugar in an easily digested form, such as orange juice, candy, or lump sugar. (M-S)

■ An unconscious patient who has hypoglycemia should receive an S.C. or I.M. injection of glucagon as prescribed by a physician or 50% dextrose by I.V. injection. (M-S)

■ A patient with diabetes mellitus should inspect his feet daily for calluses, corns, and blisters. He should also use warm water to wash his feet and trim his toenails straight across to prevent ingrown toenails. (M-S)

■ The early stage of ketoacidosis causes polyuria, polydipsia, anorexia, muscle cramps, and vomiting. The late stage causes Kussmaul's respirations, sweet breath odor, and stupor or coma. (M-S)

■ An allergen is a substance that can cause a hypersensitivity reaction. (M-S)

To maintain package sterility, the nurse should open a wrapper's top flap away from the body, open each side flap by touching only the outer part of the wrapper, and open the final flap by grasping the turned-down corner and pulling it toward the body.   **(FND)**

A corrective lens for nearsightedness is concave.   **(M-S)**

Chronic untreated hypothyroidism or abrupt withdrawal of thyroid medication may lead to myxedema coma.   **(M-S)**

Signs and symptoms of myxedema coma are lethargy, stupor, decreased level of consciousness, dry skin and hair, delayed deep tendon reflexes, progressive respiratory center depression and cerebral hypoxia, weight gain, hypothermia, and hypoglycemia.   **(M-S)**

Nearsightedness occurs when the focal point of a ray of light from an object that's 20′ (6 m) away falls in front of the retina.   **(M-S)**

Farsightedness occurs when the focal point of a ray of light from an object that's 20′ away falls behind the retina.   **(M-S)**

A corrective lens for farsightedness is convex.   **(M-S)**

Refraction is clinical measurement of the error in eye focusing.   **(M-S)**

Adhesions are bands of granulation and scar tissue that develop in some patients after a surgical incision.   **(M-S)**

The nurse should moisten an eye patch for an unconscious patient because a dry patch may irritate the cornea.   **(M-S)**

A patient who has had eye surgery shouldn't bend over, comb his hair vigorously, or engage in activity that increases intraocular pressure.   **(M-S)**

When caring for a patient who has a penetrating eye injury, the nurse should patch both eyes loosely with sterile gauze, administer an oral antibiotic (in high doses) and tetanus injection as prescribed, and refer the patient to an ophthalmologist for follow-up.   **(M-S)**

Signs and symptoms of colorectal cancer include changes in bowel habits, rectal bleeding, abdominal pain, anorexia, weight loss, malaise, anemia, and constipation or diarrhea.   **(M-S)**

When climbing stairs with crutches, the patient should lead with the uninvolved leg and follow with the crutches and involved leg.   **(M-S)**

■ When descending stairs with crutches, the patient should lead with the crutches and the involved leg and follow with the uninvolved leg. (M-S)

■ When surgery requires eyelash trimming, the nurse should apply petroleum jelly to the scissor blades so that the eyelashes will adhere to them. (M-S)

■ Pain after a corneal transplant may indicate that the dressing has been applied too tightly, the graft has slipped, or the eye is hemorrhaging. (M-S)

■ A patient with retinal detachment may report floating spots, flashes of light, and a sensation of a veil or curtain coming down. (M-S)

■ Immediate postoperative care for a patient with retinal detachment includes maintaining the eye patch and shield in place over the affected area and observing the area for drainage; maintaining the patient in the position specified by the ophthalmologist (usually, lying on his abdomen, with his head parallel to the floor and turned to the side); avoiding bumping the patient's head or bed; and encouraging deep breathing, but not coughing. (M-S)

■ A patient with a cataract may have vision disturbances, such as image distortion, light glaring, and gradual loss of vision. (M-S)

■ When talking to a hearing-impaired patient who can lip-read, the nurse should face the patient, speak slowly and enunciate clearly, point to objects as needed, and avoid chewing gum. (M-S)

■ Clinical manifestations of venous stasis ulcer include hemosiderin deposits (visible in fair-skinned individuals); dry, cracked skin; and infection. (M-S)

■ The fluorescent treponemal antibody absorption test is a specific serologic test for syphilis. (M-S)

■ To reduce fever, the nurse may give the patient a sponge bath with tepid water (80° to 93° F [26.7° to 33.9° C]). (M-S)

■ When communicating with a patient who has had a stroke, the nurse should allow ample time for the patient to speak and respond, face the patient's unaffected side, avoid talking quickly, give visual clues, supplement speech with gestures, and give instructions consistently. (M-S)

■ The major complication of Bell's palsy is keratitis (corneal inflammation), which results from incomplete eye closure on the affected side. **(M-S)**

■ Immunosuppressants are used to combat tissue rejection and help control autoimmune disorders. **(M-S)**

■ After a unilateral stroke, a patient may be able to propel a wheelchair by using a heel-to-toe movement with the unaffected leg and turning the wheel with the unaffected hand. **(M-S)**

■ First-morning urine is the most concentrated and most likely to show abnormalities. It should be refrigerated to retard bacterial growth or, for microscopic examination, should be sent to the laboratory immediately. **(M-S)**

■ A patient who is recovering from a stroke should align his arms and legs correctly, wear high-top sneakers to prevent footdrop and contracture, and use an egg crate, flotation, or pulsating mattress to help prevent pressure ulcers. **(M-S)**

■ After a fracture of the arm or leg, the bone may show complete union (normal healing), delayed union (healing that takes longer than expected), or nonunion (failure to heal). **(M-S)**

■ The most common complication of a hip fracture is thromboembolism, which may occlude an artery and cause the area it supplies to become cold and cyanotic. **(M-S)**

■ Chloral hydrate suppositories should be refrigerated. **(M-S)**

■ Cast application usually requires two persons; it shouldn't be attempted alone. **(M-S)**

■ A plaster cast reaches maximum strength in 48 hours; a synthetic cast, within 30 minutes because it doesn't require drying. **(M-S)**

■ Severe pain indicates the development of a pressure ulcer within a cast; the pain decreases significantly after the ulcer develops. **(M-S)**

■ With running traction (Buck's traction), the patient may not be turned without disrupting the line of pull. With balanced suspension traction, the patient may be elevated, turned slightly, and moved as needed. **(PED)**

■ Indications of circulatory interference are abnormal skin coolness, cyanosis, and rubor or pallor. (M-S)

■ During the postoperative phase, increasing pulse rate and decreasing blood pressure may indicate hemorrhage and impending shock. (M-S)

■ Orthopedic surgical wounds bleed more than other surgical wounds. The nurse can expect 200 to 500 ml of drainage during the first 24 hours and less than 30 ml each 8 hours for the next 48 hours. (M-S)

■ A patient who has had hip surgery shouldn't adduct or flex the affected hip because flexion greater than 90 degrees may cause dislocation. (M-S)

■ The Hoyer lift, a hydraulic device, allows two persons to lift and move a nonambulatory patient safely. (M-S)

■ A patient with carpal tunnel syndrome, a complex of symptoms caused by compression of the median nerve in the carpal tunnel, usually has weakness, pain, burning, numbness, or tingling in one or both hands. (M-S)

■ The nurse shouldn't dry a patient's ear canal or remove wax with a cotton-tipped applicator because it may force cerumen against the tympanic membrane. (FND)

■ A patient's identification bracelet should remain in place until the patient has been discharged from the health care facility and has left the premises. (FND)

■ The nurse should instruct a patient who has had heatstroke to wear light-colored, loose-fitting clothing when exposed to the sun; rest frequently; and drink plenty of fluids. (M-S)

■ A conscious patient with heat exhaustion or heatstroke should receive a solution of ½ teaspoon of salt in 120 ml of water every 15 minutes for 1 hour. (M-S)

■ An I.V. line inserted during an emergency or outside the hospital setting should be changed within 24 hours. (M-S)

■ After a tepid bath, the nurse should dry the patient thoroughly to prevent chills. (M-S)

■ The nurse should take the patient's temperature 30 minutes after completing a tepid bath.   (M-S)

■ Shower or bath water shouldn't exceed 105° F (40.6° C).   (M-S)

■ *Dilatation and curettage* is widening of the cervical canal with a dilator and scraping of the uterus with a curette.   (M-S)

■ When not in use, all central venous catheters must be capped with adaptors after flushing.   (M-S)

■ Care after dilatation and curettage consists of bed rest for 1 day, mild analgesics for pain, and use of a sterile pad for as long as bleeding persists.   (M-S)

■ If a patient feels faint during a bath or shower, the nurse should turn off the water, cover the patient, lower the patient's head, and summon help.   (M-S)

■ For the first few months of levothyroxine (Synthroid) therapy, a child may have temporary hair loss.   (PED)

■ A patient who is taking oral contraceptives shouldn't smoke because smoking can intensify the drug's adverse cardiovascular effect.   (M-S)

■ The use of soft restraints requires a physician's order and assessment and documentation of the patient and affected limbs, according to facility policy.   (M-S)

■ A vest restraint should be used cautiously in a patient with heart failure or a respiratory disorder. The restraint can tighten with movement, further limiting respiratory function. To ensure patient safety, the least amount of restraint should be used.   (M-S)

■ If a piggyback system becomes dislodged, the nurse should replace the entire piggyback system with the appropriate solution and drug, as prescribed.   (M-S)

■ The nurse shouldn't secure a restraint to a bed's side rails because they might be lowered inadvertently and cause patient injury or discomfort.   (M-S)

■ Before discharging a patient who has had an abortion, the nurse should instruct her to report bright red clots, bleeding that lasts longer than 7 days, or signs of infection, such as a temperature of greater than 100° F (37.8° C), foul-smelling vaginal discharge, severe uterine cramping, nausea, or vomiting. **(MAT)**

■ The nurse should assess a patient who has limb restraints every 30 minutes to detect signs of impaired circulation. **(M-S)**

■ The Centers for Disease Control and Prevention recommends using a needleless system for piggybacking an I.V. drug into the main I.V. line. **(M-S)**

■ When informed that a patient's amniotic membrane has broken, the nurse should check fetal heart tones and then maternal vital signs. **(MAT)**

■ If a gown is required, the nurse should put it on when she enters the patient's room and discard it when she leaves. **(M-S)**

■ When changing the dressing of a patient who is in isolation, the nurse should wear two pairs of gloves. **(M-S)**

■ The duration of pregnancy averages 280 days, 40 weeks, 9 calendar months, or 10 lunar months. **(MAT)**

■ A disposable bedpan and urinal should remain in the room of a patient who is in isolation and be discarded on discharge or at the end of the isolation period. **(M-S)**

■ Mycoses (fungal infections) may be systemic or deep (affecting the internal organs), subcutaneous (involving the skin), or superficial (growing on the outer layer of skin and hair). **(M-S)**

■ The night before a sputum specimen is to be collected by expectoration, the patient should increase fluid intake to promote sputum production. **(M-S)**

■ A sample of feces for an ova and parasite study should be collected directly into a waterproof container, covered with a lid, and sent to the laboratory immediately. If the patient is bedridden, the sample can be collected into a clean, dry bedpan and then transferred with a tongue depressor into a container. **(M-S)**

When obtaining a sputum specimen for testing, the nurse should instruct the patient to rinse his mouth with clean water, cough deeply from his chest, and expectorate into a sterile container.   **(M-S)**

Tonometry allows indirect measurement of intraocular pressure and aids in early detection of glaucoma.   **(M-S)**

Pulmonary function tests (a series of measurements that evaluate ventilatory function through spirometric measurements) help to diagnose pulmonary dysfunction.   **(M-S)**

After a liver biopsy, the patient should lie on the right side to compress the biopsy site and decrease the possibility of bleeding.   **(M-S)**

A patient who has cirrhosis should follow a diet that restricts sodium, but provides protein and vitamins (especially B, C, and K, and folate).   **(M-S)**

If 12 hours of gastric suction don't relieve bowel obstruction, surgery is indicated.   **(M-S)**

The nurse can puncture a nifedipine (Procardia) capsule with a needle, withdraw its liquid, and instill it into the buccal pouch.   **(M-S)**

When administering whole blood or packed red blood cells (RBCs), the nurse should use a 16 to 20G needle or cannula to avoid RBC hemolysis.   **(M-S)**

Hirsutism is excessive body hair in a masculine distribution.   **(M-S)**

The Controlled Substances Act designated five categories, or schedules, that classify controlled drugs according to their abuse potential.   **(FND)**

Schedule I drugs, such as heroin, have a high abuse potential and have no currently accepted medical use in the United States.   **(FND)**

Schedule II drugs, such as morphine, opium, and meperidine (Demerol), have a high abuse potential, but currently have accepted medical uses. Their use may lead to physical or psychological dependence.   **(FND)**

Schedule III drugs, such as paregoric and butabarbital (Butisol), have a lower abuse potential than Schedule I or II drugs. Abuse of Schedule III drugs may lead to moderate or low physical or psychological dependence, or both.   **(FND)**

▓ Schedule IV drugs, such as chloral hydrate, have a low abuse potential compared with Schedule III drugs.   **(FND)**

▓ Schedule V drugs, such as cough syrups that contain codeine, have the lowest abuse potential of the controlled substances.   **(FND)**

▓ One unit of whole blood or packed red blood cells is administered over 2 to 4 hours.   **(M-S)**

▓ To administer an I.V. drug in an infant or an older patient with small veins, the nurse should use a 21G or 23G winged set, dilute the drug as prescribed, and infuse it slowly to prevent vein injury.   **(PED)**

▓ Scurvy is associated with vitamin C deficiency.   **(M-S)**

▓ A *vitamin* is an organic compound that usually can't be synthesized by the body and is needed in metabolic processes.   **(M-S)**

▓ An adolescent's eating habits are significantly influenced by his peer group.   **(PED)**

▓ In an infant, hypothyroidism causes inactivity, excessive sleeping, and minimal crying. The infant may be described as a "good baby."   **(PED)**

▓ Pulmonary embolism can be caused when thromboembolism of fat, blood, bone marrow, or amniotic fluid obstructs the pulmonary artery.   **(M-S)**

▓ After maxillofacial surgery, a patient whose mandible and maxilla have been wired together should keep a pair of scissors or wire cutters readily available so that he can cut the wires and prevent aspiration if vomiting occurs.   **(M-S)**

▓ Rapid instillation of fluid during colonic irrigation can cause abdominal cramping.   **(M-S)**

▓ A collaborative relationship between health care workers helps shorten the hospital stay and increases patient satisfaction.   **(M-S)**

▓ For elderly patients in a health care facility, predictable hazards include nighttime confusion (sundowning), fractures from falling, immobility-induced pressure ulcers, prolonged convalescence, and loss of home and support systems.   **(M-S)**

- Respiratory tract infections, especially viral infections, can trigger asthma attacks. (M-S)

- Oxygen therapy is used in severe asthma attacks to prevent or treat hypoxemia. (M-S)

- During an asthma attack, the patient may prefer nasal prongs to a Venturi mask because of the mask's smothering effect. (M-S)

- Chronic obstructive pulmonary disease usually develops over a period of years. In 95% of patients, it results from smoking. (M-S)

- An early sign of chronic obstructive pulmonary disease (COPD) is slowing of forced expiration. A healthy person can empty the lungs in less than 4 seconds; a patient with COPD may take 6 to 10 seconds. (M-S)

- Chronic obstructive pulmonary disease eventually leads to structural changes in the lungs, including overdistended alveoli and hyperinflated lungs. (M-S)

- Cystic fibrosis, which is transmitted as an autosomal recessive trait, causes dysfunction of the exocrine gland, sweat glands, and respiratory and digestive systems. (PED)

- In the neonate, a common manifestation of cystic fibrosis is meconium ileus caused by obstruction of the small intestine by viscous meconium. (PED)

- Neonates who have cystic fibrosis but don't have meconium ileus at birth have good appetites, but gain weight slowly. (PED)

- Cellulitis causes localized heat, redness, swelling and, occasionally, fever, chills, and malaise. (M-S)

- The initial weight loss for a healthy neonate is 5% to 10% of birth weight. (MAT)

- The normal hemoglobin value in neonates is 17 to 20 g/dl. (MAT)

- Venous stasis may precipitate thrombophlebitis. (M-S)

- Treatment of thrombophlebitis includes leg elevation, heat application, and possibly, anticoagulant therapy. (M-S)

- A suctioning machine should remain at the bedside of a patient who has had maxillofacial surgery. (M-S)

- For a bedridden patient with heart failure, the nurse should check for edema in the sacral area.   (M-S)

- *Crowning* is the appearance of the fetus's head when its largest diameter is encircled by the vulvovaginal ring.   (MAT)

- If an immunization schedule is interrupted, it should be restarted from the last immunization administered, not from the beginning.   (PED)

- In passive range-of-motion exercises, the therapist moves the patient's joints through as full a range of motion as possible to improve or maintain joint mobility and help prevent contractures.   (M-S)

- In resistance exercises, which allow muscle length to change, the patient performs exercises against resistance applied by the therapist.   (M-S)

- In isometric exercises, the patient contracts muscles against stable resistance, but without joint movement. Muscle length remains the same, but strength and tone may increase.   (M-S)

- *Impetigo* is a contagious, superficial, vesicopustular skin infection. Predisposing factors include poor hygiene, anemia, malnutrition, and a warm climate.   (M-S)

- *Activities of daily living* are actions that the patient must perform every day to provide self-care and to interact with society.   (FND)

- After cardiopulmonary resuscitation (CPR) begins, it shouldn't be interrupted, except when the administrator is alone and must summon help. In this case, the administrator should perform CPR for 1 minute before calling for help.   (M-S)

- The tongue is the most common airway obstruction in an unconscious patient.   (M-S)

- For adult cardiopulmonary resuscitation, the chest compression rate is 80 to 100 times per minute.   (M-S)

- A patient with ulcers should avoid bedtime snacks because food may stimulate nocturnal secretions.   (M-S)

- In angioplasty, a blood vessel is dilated with a balloon catheter that's inserted through the skin and the vessel's lumen to the narrowed area. Once in place, the balloon is inflated to flatten plaque against the vessel wall.   (M-S)

A full liquid diet supplies nutrients, fluids, and calories in simple, easily digested foods, such as apple juice, cream of wheat, milk, coffee, strained cream soup, high-protein gelatin, cranberry juice, custard, and ice cream. It's prescribed for patients who can't tolerate a regular diet.   (M-S)

A pureed diet meets the patient's nutritional needs without including foods that are difficult to chew or swallow. Food is blended to a semi-solid consistency.   (M-S)

A soft, or light, diet is specifically designed for patients who have difficulty chewing or tolerating a regular diet. It's nutritionally adequate and consists of foods such as orange juice, cream of wheat, scrambled eggs, enriched toast, cream of chicken soup, wheat bread, fruit cocktail, and mushroom soup.   (M-S)

A regular diet is provided for patients who don't require dietary modification.   (M-S)

A pediatric diet is normally ordered as "diet for age" by the physician. It should include sufficient nutrients and calories to promote growth and development.   (PED)

A bland diet restricts foods that cause gastric irritation or produce acid secretion without providing a neutralizing effect.   (M-S)

A clear liquid diet provides fluid and a gradual return to a regular diet. This type of diet is deficient in all nutrients and should be followed for only a short period.   (M-S)

Patients with a gastric ulcer should avoid alcohol, caffeinated beverages, aspirin, and spicy foods.   (M-S)

In active assistance exercises, the patient performs exercises with the therapist's help.   (M-S)

Penicillinase is an enzyme produced by certain bacteria. It converts penicillin into an inactive product, increasing the bacteria's resistance to the antibiotic.   (M-S)

Battle's sign is a bluish discoloration behind the ear in some patients who sustain a basilar skull fracture.   (M-S)

Crackles are nonmusical clicking or rattling noises that are heard during auscultation of abnormal breath sounds. They are caused by air passing through fluid-filled airways.   (M-S)

▓ Antibiotics aren't effective against viruses, protozoa, or parasites. (M-S)

▓ Most penicillins and cephalosporins produce their antibiotic effects by cell wall inhibition. (M-S)

▓ When assessing a patient with an inguinal hernia, the nurse should suspect strangulation if the patient reports severe pain, nausea, and vomiting. (M-S)

▓ *Phimosis* is tightness of the prepuce of the penis that prevents retraction of the foreskin over the glans. (M-S)

▓ *Aminoglycosides* are natural antibiotics that are effective against gram-negative bacteria. They must be used with caution because they can cause nephrotoxicity and ototoxicity. (M-S)

▓ On scrotal examination, varicoceles and tumors don't transilluminate, but spermatoceles and hydroceles do. (M-S)

▓ The heart of a child with tetralogy of Fallot appears boot-shaped on X-ray films because the right ventricle is enlarged. (PED)

▓ Testing of the six cardinal fields of gaze evaluates the function of all extraocular muscles and cranial nerves III, IV, and VI. (FND)

▓ A *hordeolum* (eyelid stye) is an infection of one or more sebaceous glands of the eyelid. (M-S)

▓ A *chalazion* is an eyelid mass that's caused by chronic inflammation of the meibomian gland. (M-S)

▓ During ophthalmoscopic examination, the absence of the red reflex indicates a lens opacity (cataract) or a detached retina. (M-S)

▓ Respiratory acidosis is associated with conditions such as drug overdose, Guillain-Barré syndrome, myasthenia gravis, chronic obstructive pulmonary disease, pickwickian syndrome, and kyphoscoliosis. (M-S)

▓ Respiratory alkalosis is associated with conditions such as high fever, severe hypoxia, asthma, and pulmonary embolism. (M-S)

▓ Metabolic acidosis is associated with such conditions as renal failure, diarrhea, diabetic ketosis, and lactic ketosis, and with high doses of acetazolamide (Diamox). (M-S)

Gastrectomy is surgical excision of all or part of the stomach to remove a chronic peptic ulcer, stop hemorrhage in a perforated ulcer, or remove a malignant tumor.   (M-S)

Metabolic alkalosis is associated with nasogastric suctioning, excessive use of diuretics, and steroid therapy.   (M-S)

Vitiligo (a benign, acquired skin disease) is marked by stark white skin patches that are caused by the destruction and loss of pigment cells.
                                                                                (M-S)

A *multipara* is a woman who has had two or more pregnancies that progressed to viability, regardless of whether the offspring were alive at birth.
                                                                                (MAT)

Overdose or accidental overingestion of disulfiram (Antabuse) should be treated with gastric aspiration or lavage and supportive therapy.
                                                                                (M-S)

The six types of heart murmurs are graded from 1 to 6. A grade 6 heart murmur can be heard with the stethoscope slightly raised from the chest.
                                                                                (FND)

The causes of abdominal distention are represented by the six F's: flatus, feces, fetus, fluid, fat, and fatal (malignant) neoplasm.   (M-S)

A positive Murphy's sign indicates cholecystitis.   (M-S)

Signs of appendicitis include right abdominal pain, abdominal rigidity and rebound tenderness, nausea, and anorexia.   (M-S)

Ascites can be detected when more than 500 ml of fluid has collected in the intraperitoneal space.   (M-S)

The most important goal to include in a care plan is the patient's goal.
                                                                                (FND)

For a patient with organic brain syndrome or a senile disease, the ideal environment is stable and limits confusion.   (M-S)

In a patient with organic brain syndrome, memory loss usually affects all spheres, but begins with recent memory loss.   (M-S)

In a pregnant patient, preeclampsia may progress to eclampsia, which is characterized by seizures and may lead to coma.   (MAT)

The Apgar score is used to assess the neonate's vital functions. It's obtained at 1 minute and 5 minutes after delivery. The score is based on respiratory effort, heart rate, muscle tone, reflex irritability, and color.
(MAT)

During cardiac catheterization, the patient may experience a thudding sensation in the chest, a strong desire to cough, and a transient feeling of heat, usually in the face, as a result of injection of the contrast medium.
(M-S)

Because of the anti-insulin effects of placental hormones, insulin requirements increase during the third trimester.   (MAT)

Gestational age can be estimated by ultrasound measurement of maternal abdominal circumference, fetal femur length, and fetal head size. These measurements are most accurate between 12 and 18 weeks' gestation.   (MAT)

Skeletal system abnormalities and ventricular septal defects are the most common disorders of infants who are born to diabetic women. The incidence of congenital malformation is three times higher in these infants than in those born to nondiabetic women.   (MAT)

Slight bubbling in the suction column of a thoracic drainage system, such as a Pleur-evac unit, indicates that the system is working properly. A lack of bubbling in the suction chamber indicates inadequate suction. (M-S)

Nutritional deficiency is a common finding in people who have a long history of alcohol abuse.   (M-S)

Treatment for alcohol withdrawal may include administration of I.V. glucose for hypoglycemia, I.V. fluid containing thiamine and other B vitamins, and antianxiety, antidiarrheal, anticonvulsant, and antiemetic drugs.   (PSY)

The alcoholic patient receives thiamine to help prevent peripheral neuropathy and Korsakoff's syndrome.   (PSY)

Alcohol withdrawal may precipitate seizure activity because alcohol lowers the seizure threshold in some people.   (PSY)

Paraphrasing is an active listening technique in which the nurse restates what the patient has just said.   (PSY)

■ A patient with Korsakoff's syndrome may use confabulation (made up information) to cover memory lapses or periods of amnesia.   **(PSY)**

■ In the patient with varicose veins, graduated compression elastic stockings (30 to 40 mm Hg) may be prescribed to promote venous return.
(M-S)

■ Nonviral hepatitis usually results from exposure to certain chemicals or drugs.   **(M-S)**

■ The patient with preeclampsia usually has puffiness around the eyes or edema in the hands (for example, "I can't put my wedding ring on.").
(MAT)

■ Substantial elevation of the serum transaminase level is a symptom of acute hepatitis.   **(M-S)**

■ Normal cardiac output is 4 to 6 L/minute, with a stroke volume of 60 to 70 ml.   **(M-S)**

■ Excessive vomiting or removal of the stomach contents through suction can decrease the potassium level and lead to hypokalemia.   **(M-S)**

■ As a heparin antagonist, protamine is an antidote for heparin overdose.
(M-S)

■ People with obsessive-compulsive disorder realize that their behavior is unreasonable, but are powerless to control it.   **(PSY)**

■ If a patient has a positive reaction to a tuberculin skin test, such as the purified protein derivative test, the nurse should suspect current or past exposure. The nurse should ask the patient about a history of tuberculosis (TB) and the presence of early signs and symptoms of TB, such as low-grade fever, weight loss, night sweats, fatigue, and anorexia.   **(M-S)**

■ Signs and symptoms of acute rheumatic fever include chorea, fever, carditis, migratory polyarthritis, erythema marginatum (rash), and subcutaneous nodules.   **(M-S)**

■ Before undergoing any invasive dental procedure, the patient who has a history of rheumatic fever should receive prophylactic penicillin therapy. This therapy helps to prevent contamination of the blood with oral bacteria, which could migrate to the heart valves.   **(M-S)**

■ Fruits are high in fiber and low in protein, and should be omitted from a low-residue diet. **(FND)**

■ The nurse should use an objective scale to assess and quantify pain. Postoperative pain varies greatly among individuals. **(FND)**

■ After a myocardial infarction, most patients can resume sexual activity when they can climb two flights of stairs without fatigue or dyspnea. **(M-S)**

■ Elderly patients are susceptible to orthostatic hypotension because the baroreceptors become less sensitive to position changes as people age. **(M-S)**

■ Kegel exercises require contraction and relaxation of the perineal muscles. These exercises help strengthen pelvic muscles and improve urine control in postpartum patients. **(MAT)**

■ When witnessing psychiatric patients who are engaged in a threatening confrontation, the nurse should first separate the two individuals. **(PSY)**

■ Symptoms of postpartum depression range from mild postpartum blues to intense, suicidal, depressive psychosis. **(MAT)**

■ The preterm neonate may require gavage feedings because of a weak sucking reflex, uncoordinated sucking, or respiratory distress. **(MAT)**

■ Postmortem care includes cleaning and preparing the deceased patient for family viewing, arranging transportation to the morgue or funeral home, and determining the disposition of belongings. **(FND)**

■ For the patient with suspected renal or urethral calculi, the nurse should strain the urine to determine whether calculi have been passed. **(M-S)**

■ The nurse should place the patient with ascites in the semi-Fowler position because it permits maximum lung expansion. **(M-S)**

■ For the patient who has ingested poison, the nurse should save the vomitus for analysis. **(M-S)**

■ The nurse should provide honest answers to the patient's questions. **(FND)**

Acrocyanosis (blueness and coolness of the arms and legs) is normal in neonates because of their immature peripheral circulatory system.

(MAT)

The earliest signs of respiratory distress are increased respiratory rate and increased pulse rate. (M-S)

In adults, gastroenteritis is commonly self-limiting and causes diarrhea, abdominal discomfort, nausea, and vomiting. (M-S)

Cardiac output equals stroke volume multiplied by the heart rate per minute. (M-S)

Milk shouldn't be included in a clear liquid diet. (FND)

In patients with acute meningitis, the cerebrospinal fluid protein level is elevated. (M-S)

When a patient is suspected of having food poisoning, the nurse should notify public health authorities so that they can interview patients and food handlers and take samples of the suspected contaminated food.

(M-S)

The patient who is receiving a potassium-wasting diuretic should eat potassium-rich foods. (M-S)

When caring for an infant, a child, or a confused patient, consistency in nursing personnel is paramount. (FND)

A patient with chronic obstructive pulmonary disease should receive low-level oxygen administration by nasal cannula (2 to 3 L/minute) to avoid interfering with the hypoxic drive. (M-S)

The hypothalamus secretes vasopressin and oxytocin, which are stored in the pituitary gland. (FND)

The three membranes that enclose the brain and spinal cord are the dura mater, pia mater, and arachnoid. (FND)

A nasogastric tube is used to remove fluid and gas from the small intestine preoperatively or postoperatively. (FND)

To prevent ophthalmia neonatorum (a severe eye infection caused by maternal gonorrhea), the nurse may administer one of three drugs, as prescribed, in the neonate's eyes: tetracycline, silver nitrate, or erythromycin. (MAT)

■ In metabolic acidosis, the patient may have Kussmaul's respirations because the rate and depth of respirations increase to "blow off" excess carbonic acids. **(M-S)**

■ In women, gonorrhea affects the vagina and fallopian tubes. **(M-S)**

■ Phenylketonuria is an inborn error of phenylalanine metabolism that causes high serum levels of phenylalanine that might lead to cerebral damage and mental retardation. **(PED)**

■ After traumatic amputation, the greatest threats to the patient are blood loss and hypovolemic shock. Initial interventions should control bleeding and replace fluid and blood as needed. **(M-S)**

■ Epinephrine is a sympathomimetic drug that acts primarily on alpha, beta$_1$, and beta$_2$ receptors, causing vasoconstriction. **(M-S)**

■ Epinephrine's adverse effects include dyspnea, tachycardia, palpitations, headaches, and hypertension. **(M-S)**

■ Psychologists, physical therapists, and chiropractors aren't authorized to write prescriptions for drugs. **(FND)**

■ The area around a stoma is cleaned with mild soap and water. **(FND)**

■ Vegetables have a high fiber content. **(FND)**

■ A cardinal sign of pancreatitis is an elevated serum amylase level. **(M-S)**

■ High colonic irrigation is used to stimulate peristalsis and reduce flatulence. **(M-S)**

■ The nurse should use a tuberculin syringe to administer a subcutaneous injection of less than 1 ml. **(FND)**

■ Bleeding is the most common postoperative problem. **(M-S)**

■ The patient can control some colostomy odors by avoiding such foods as fish, eggs, onions, beans, and cabbage and related vegetables. **(M-S)**

■ For adults, subcutaneous injections require a 25G 1″ needle; for infants, children, elderly, or very thin patients, they require a 25G to 27G ½″ needle. **(FND)**

■ Before administering a drug, the nurse should identify the patient by checking the identification band and asking the patient to state his name. **(FND)**

- To clean the skin before an injection, the nurse uses a sterile alcohol swab to wipe from the center of the site outward in a circular motion. (FND)

- The nurse should inject heparin deep into subcutaneous tissue at a 90-degree angle (perpendicular to the skin) to prevent skin irritation. (FND)

- If blood is aspirated into the syringe before an I.M. injection, the nurse should withdraw the needle, prepare another syringe, and repeat the procedure. (FND)

- The nurse shouldn't cut the patient's hair without written consent from the patient or an appropriate relative. (FND)

- If bleeding occurs after an injection, the nurse should apply pressure until the bleeding stops. If bruising occurs, the nurse should monitor the site for an enlarging hematoma. (FND)

- When providing hair and scalp care, the nurse should begin combing at the end of the hair and work toward the head. (FND)

- The frequency of patient hair care depends on the length and texture of the hair, the duration of hospitalization, and the patient's condition. (FND)

- When paralysis or coma impairs or erases the corneal reflex, frequent eye care is performed to keep the exposed cornea moist, preventing ulceration and inflammation. (M-S)

- Proper function of a hearing aid requires careful handling during insertion and removal, regular cleaning of the ear piece to prevent wax buildup, and prompt replacement of dead batteries. (FND)

- The hearing aid that's marked with a blue dot is for the left ear; the one with a red dot is for the right ear. (FND)

- A hearing aid shouldn't be exposed to heat or humidity and shouldn't be immersed in water. (FND)

- The nurse should instruct the patient to avoid using hair spray while wearing a hearing aid. (FND)

- The five branches of pharmacology are pharmacokinetics, pharmacodynamics, pharmacotherapeutics, toxicology, and pharmacognosy. (FND)

■ Interventions for the patient with acquired immunodeficiency syndrome include treating existing infections and cancers, reducing the risk of opportunistic infections, maintaining adequate nutrition and hydration, and providing emotional support to the patient and family.   (M-S)

■ The nurse should remove heel protectors every 8 hours to inspect the foot for signs of skin breakdown.   (FND)

■ Signs and symptoms of chlamydial infection are urinary frequency; thin, white vaginal or urethral discharge; and cervical inflammation.   (M-S)

■ Heat is applied to promote vasodilation, which reduces pain caused by inflammation.   (FND)

■ Chlamydial infection is the most prevalent sexually transmitted disease in the United States.   (M-S)

■ The pituitary gland is located in the sella turcica of the sphenoid bone in the cranial cavity.   (M-S)

■ *Myasthenia gravis* is a neuromuscular disorder that's characterized by impulse disturbances at the myoneural junction.   (M-S)

■ A sutured surgical incision is an example of healing by first intention (healing directly, without granulation).   (FND)

■ Healing by secondary intention (healing by granulation) is closure of the wound when granulation tissue fills the defect and allows reepithelialization to occur, beginning at the wound edges and continuing to the center, until the entire wound is covered.   (FND)

■ Keloid formation is an abnormality in healing that's characterized by overgrowth of scar tissue at the wound site.   (FND)

■ Patients with anorexia nervosa or bulimia must be observed during meals and for some time afterward to ensure that they don't purge what they have eaten.   (PSY)

■ Myasthenia gravis, which usually affects young women, causes extreme muscle weakness and fatigability, difficulty chewing and talking, strabismus, and ptosis.   (M-S)

■ Transsexuals believe that they were born the wrong gender and may seek hormonal or surgical treatment to change their gender.   (PSY)

Tay-Sachs disease is caused by a congenital enzyme deficiency and is characterized by progressive mental and motor deterioration and cherry-red spots on the macula. **(PED)**

Hypothermia is a life-threatening disorder in which the body's core temperature drops below 95° F (35° C). **(M-S)**

To prevent brain damage, treatment of phenylketonuria must begin within the first few weeks of life. **(PED)**

Neonatal testing for phenylketonuria is mandatory in most states. **(MAT)**

Although no cure exists for Tay-Sachs disease, serum analysis for hexosaminidase A deficiency allows accurate identification of genetic carriers of the disease. **(PED)**

Signs and symptoms of hypopituitarism in adults may include gonadal failure, diabetes insipidus, hypothyroidism, and adrenocortical insufficiency. **(M-S)**

Reiter's syndrome causes a triad of symptoms: arthritis, conjunctivitis, and urethritis. **(M-S)**

Down syndrome (trisomy 21) is the most common chromosomal disorder. **(PED)**

For patients who have had a partial gastrectomy, a carbohydrate-restricted diet includes foods that are high in protein and fats and restricts foods that are high in carbohydrates. High-carbohydrate foods are digested quickly and are readily emptied from the stomach into the duodenum, causing diarrhea and dumping syndrome. **(M-S)**

The nurse should place the neonate in a 30-degree Trendelenburg position to facilitate mucus drainage. **(MAT)**

The nurse may suction the neonate's nose and mouth as needed with a bulb syringe or suction trap. **(MAT)**

To prevent heat loss, the nurse should place the neonate under a radiant warmer during suctioning and initial delivery-room care, and then wrap the neonate in a warmed blanket for transport to the nursery. **(MAT)**

The umbilical cord normally has two arteries and one vein. **(MAT)**

When providing care, the nurse should expose only one part of an infant's body at a time. **(MAT)**

▓ *Lightening* is settling of the fetal head into the brim of the pelvis. (MAT)

▓ If the neonate is stable, the mother should be allowed to breast-feed within the neonate's first hour of life.   (MAT)

▓ The nurse should check the neonate's temperature every 1 to 2 hours until it's maintained within normal limits.   (MAT)

▓ At birth, a neonate normally weighs 5 to 9 lb (2 to 4 kg), measures 18" to 22" (45.5 to 56 cm) in length, has a head circumference of 13½" to 14" (34 to 35.5 cm), and has a chest circumference that's 1" (2.5 cm) less than the head circumference.   (MAT)

▓ In the neonate, temperature normally ranges from 98° to 99° F (36.7° to 37.2° C), apical pulse rate averages 120 to 160 beats/minute, and respirations are 40 to 60 breaths/minute.   (MAT)

▓ The diamond-shaped anterior fontanel usually closes between ages 12 and 18 months. The triangular posterior fontanel usually closes by age 2 months.   (MAT)

▓ In the neonate, a straight spine is normal. A tuft of hair over the spine is an abnormal finding.   (MAT)

▓ Prostaglandin gel may be applied to the vagina or cervix to ripen an unfavorable cervix before labor induction with oxytocin (Pitocin). (MAT)

▓ When administering an oral drug to an infant, the nurse should place it in the side of the mouth and encourage swallowing by gently lifting the infant's chin with the thumb and stroking the infant's neck.

(PED)

▓ Supernumerary nipples are occasionally seen on neonates. They usually appear along a line that runs from each axilla, through the normal nipple area, and to the groin.   (MAT)

▓ *Meconium* is a material that collects in the fetus's intestines and forms the neonate's first feces, which are black and tarry.   (MAT)

▓ The presence of meconium in the amniotic fluid during labor indicates possible fetal distress and the need to evaluate the neonate for meconium aspiration.   (MAT)

▓ Polydactyly (more than the normal number of fingers or toes) is a congenital anomaly.   (PED)

A positive Babinski's reflex (toe fanning when the sole is stroked from heel to toe) is normal in the neonate and may persist for up to 18 months. **(PED)**

To assess a neonate's rooting reflex, the nurse touches a finger to the cheek or the corner of the mouth. Normally, the neonate turns his head toward the stimulus, opens his mouth, and searches for the stimulus. **(MAT)**

Harlequin sign is present when a neonate who is lying on his side appears red on the dependent side and pale on the upper side. **(MAT)**

The nurse should administer procaine penicillin by deep I.M. injection in the upper outer portion of the buttocks in the adult or in the midlateral thigh in the child. The nurse shouldn't massage the injection site. **(FND)**

Mongolian spots can range from brown to blue. Their color depends on how close melanocytes are to the surface of the skin. They most commonly appear as patches across the sacrum, buttocks, and legs. **(MAT)**

Mongolian spots are common in non-white infants and usually disappear by age 2 to 3 years. **(MAT)**

Vernix caseosa is a cheeselike substance that covers and protects the fetus's skin in utero. It may be rubbed into the neonate's skin or washed away in one or two baths. **(MAT)**

Fugue is a dissociative state in which a person leaves his familiar surroundings, assumes a new identity, and has amnesia about his previous identity. (It's also described as "flight from himself.") **(PSY)**

Caput succedaneum is edema that develops in and under the fetal scalp during labor and delivery. It resolves spontaneously and presents no danger to the neonate. The edema doesn't cross the suture line. **(MAT)**

Nevus flammeus, or port-wine stain, is a diffuse pink to dark bluish red lesion on a neonate's face or neck. **(MAT)**

Strawberry hemangiomas are raised, red birthmarks that may continue to spread up to age 1 year. Complete shrinkage and absorption of hemangiomas may take 7 to 10 years. **(PED)**

Cavernous hemangiomas resemble strawberry hemangiomas, but don't disappear with age. **(PED)**

■ The Guthrie test (a screening test for phenylketonuria) is most reliable if it's done between the second and sixth days after birth and is performed after the neonate has ingested protein. (MAT)

■ To assess coordination of sucking and swallowing, the nurse should observe the neonate's first breast-feeding or sterile water bottle-feeding. (MAT)

■ To establish a milk supply pattern, the mother should breast-feed her infant at least every 4 hours. During the first month, she should breast-feed 8 to 12 times daily (demand feeding). (MAT)

■ To avoid contact with blood and other body fluids, the nurse should wear gloves when handling the neonate until after the first bath is given. (MAT)

■ For the infant with a suspected infection, the nurse should maintain isolation and take other appropriate precautions. (PED)

■ If a breast-fed infant is content, has good skin turgor, an adequate number of wet diapers, and normal weight gain, the mother's milk supply is assumed to be adequate. (MAT)

■ A woman of childbearing age who is undergoing chemotherapy should be encouraged to use a contraceptive because of the risk of fetal damage if she becomes pregnant. (M-S)

■ *Pernicious anemia* is vitamin B_{12} deficiency that's caused by a lack of intrinsic factor, which is produced by the gastric mucosal parietal cells. (M-S)

■ To perform pursed-lip breathing, the patient inhales through the nose and exhales slowly and evenly against pursed lips while contracting the abdominal muscles. (M-S)

■ An ascending colostomy drains fluid feces. A descending colostomy drains solid fecal matter. (FND)

■ A patient who is undergoing chemotherapy should consume a high-calorie, high-protein diet. (M-S)

■ Adverse effects of chemotherapy include bone marrow depression, which causes anemia, leukopenia, and thrombocytopenia; GI epithelial cell irritation, which causes GI ulceration, bleeding, and vomiting; and destruction of hair follicles and skin, which causes alopecia and dermatitis. (M-S)

An infant with celiac disease has fatty, foul-smelling feces.   (PED)

The hemoglobin electrophoresis test differentiates between sickle cell trait and sickle cell anemia.   (M-S)

A folded towel (scrotal bridge) can provide scrotal support for the patient with scrotal edema caused by vasectomy, epididymitis, or orchitis.   (FND)

In the supine position, a pregnant patient's enlarged uterus impairs venous return from the lower half of the body to the heart, resulting in supine hypotensive syndrome, or inferior vena cava syndrome.   (MAT)

Treatment of ankle edema in the pregnant patient consists of frequent periods of rest, elevation of the foot, and avoidance of constrictive clothing, such as garters and panty hose.   (MAT)

The antibiotics erythromycin, clindamycin, and tetracycline act by inhibiting protein synthesis in susceptible organisms.   (M-S)

Eruption is the normal presentation of a tooth as it penetrates the gum.   (PED)

The nurse administers oxygen as prescribed to the patient with heart failure to help overcome hypoxia and dyspnea.   (M-S)

Signs and symptoms of small-bowel obstruction include decreased or absent bowel sounds, abdominal distention, decreased flatus, and projectile vomiting.   (M-S)

The nurse should use both hands when ventilating a patient with a manual resuscitation bag. One hand can deliver only 400 cc of air; two hands can deliver 1,000 cc of air.   (M-S)

Dosages of methylxanthine agents, such as theophylline (Theo-Dur) and aminophylline (Aminophyllin), should be individualized based on serum drug level, patient response, and adverse reactions.   (M-S)

When determining which information to give a hospitalized child about a procedure, the nurse should consider the child's developmental age, not his chronological age.   (PED)

The patient should apply a transdermal scopolamine patch (Transderm-Scop) at least 4 hours before its antiemetic action is needed.   (M-S)

- Early indications of gangrene are edema, pain, redness, darkening of the tissue, and coldness in the affected body part. (M-S)

- Ipecac syrup is the emetic of choice because of its effectiveness in evacuating the stomach and relatively low incidence of adverse reactions. (M-S)

- When giving an injection to a patient who has a bleeding disorder, the nurse should use a small-gauge needle and apply pressure to the site for 5 minutes after the injection. (FND)

- *Platelets* are the smallest and most fragile formed element of the blood and are essential for coagulation. (FND)

- To insert a nasogastric tube, the nurse instructs the patient to tilt the head back slightly and then inserts the tube. When the nurse feels the tube curving at the pharynx, the nurse should tell the patient to tilt the head forward to close the trachea and open the esophagus by swallowing. (Sips of water can facilitate this action.) (FND)

- Oral iron (ferrous sulfate) may cause green to black feces. (M-S)

- Polycythemia vera causes pruritus, painful fingers and toes, hyperuricemia, plethora (reddish purple skin and mucosa), weakness, and easy fatigability. (M-S)

- Rheumatic fever is usually preceded by a group A beta-hemolytic streptococcal infection, such as scarlet fever, otitis media, streptococcal throat infection, impetigo, or tonsillitis. (M-S)

- A *thyroid storm*, or crisis, is an extreme form of hyperthyroidism. It's characterized by hyperpyrexia with a temperature of up to 106° F (41.1° C), diarrhea, dehydration, tachycardia of up to 200 beats/minute, arrhythmias, extreme irritability, hypotension, and delirium. It may lead to coma, shock, and death. (M-S)

- Tardive dyskinesia, an adverse reaction to long-term use of antipsychotic drugs, causes involuntary repetitive movements of the tongue, lips, extremities, and trunk. (M-S)

- Tocolytic agents used to treat preterm labor include terbutaline (Brethine), ritodrine (Yutopar), and magnesium sulfate. (MAT)

- A pregnant woman who has hyperemesis gravidarum may require hospitalization to treat dehydration and starvation. (MAT)

Asthma is bronchoconstriction in response to allergens, such as food, pollen, and drugs; irritants, such as smoke and paint fumes; infections; weather changes; exercise; or gastroesophageal reflux. In the United States, about 5% of children have chronic asthma.　(M-S)

Diaphragmatic hernia is one of the most urgent neonatal surgical emergencies. By compressing and displacing the lungs and heart, this disorder can cause respiratory distress shortly after birth.　(MAT)

Blood cultures help identify the cause of endocarditis. An increased white blood cell count suggests bacterial infection.　(M-S)

Common complications of early pregnancy (up to 20 weeks' gestation) include fetal loss and serious threats to maternal health.　(MAT)

In a patient who has acute aortic dissection, the nursing priority is to maintain the mean arterial pressure between 60 and 65 mm Hg. A vasodilator such as nitroprusside (Nitropress) may be needed to achieve this goal.　(M-S)

For a patient with heart failure, one of the most important nursing diagnoses is *Decreased cardiac output related to altered myocardial contractility, increased preload and afterload, and altered rate, rhythm, or electrical conduction.*　(M-S)

For a patient receiving peritoneal dialysis, the nurse must monitor body weight and blood urea nitrogen, creatinine, and electrolyte levels. (M-S)

Angiotensin-converting enzyme inhibitors, such as captopril (Capoten) and enalapril (Vasotec), decrease blood pressure by interfering with the renin-angiotensin-aldosterone system.　(M-S)

A patient who has stable ventricular tachycardia has a blood pressure and is conscious; therefore, the patient's cardiac output is being maintained, and the nurse must monitor the patient's vital signs continuously.(M-S)

Angiotensin-converting enzyme inhibitors inhibit the enzyme that converts angiotensin I into angiotensin II, which is a potent vasoconstrictor. Through this action, they reduce peripheral arterial resistance and blood pressure.　(M-S)

In a patient who is receiving a diuretic, the nurse should monitor serum electrolyte levels, check vital signs, and observe for orthostatic hypotension.　(M-S)

▓ Families with loved ones in intensive care units report that their four most important needs are to have their questions answered honestly, to be assured that the best possible care is being provided, to know the patient's prognosis, and to feel that there is hope of recovery.   **(FND)**

▓ Breast self-examination is one of the most important health habits to teach a woman. It should be performed 1 week after the menstrual period because that's when hormonal effects, which can cause breast lumps and tenderness, are reduced.   **(M-S)**

▓ Postmenopausal women should choose a regular time each month to perform breast self-examination (for example, on the same day of the month as the woman's birthday).   **(M-S)**

▓ The difference between acute and chronic arterial disease is that the acute disease process is life-threatening.   **(M-S)**

▓ When preparing the patient for chest tube removal, the nurse should explain that removal may cause pain or a burning or pulling sensation.

(M-S)

▓ Essential hypertensive renal disease is commonly characterized by progressive renal impairment.   **(M-S)**

▓ Fetal embodiment is a maternal developmental task that occurs in the second trimester. During this stage, the mother may complain that she never gets to sleep because the fetus always gives her a thump when she tries.   **(MAT)**

▓ *Visualization* in pregnancy is a process in which the mother imagines what the child she's carrying is like and becomes acquainted with it.   **(MAT)**

▓ Mean arterial pressure (MAP) is calculated using the following formula, where S = systolic pressure and D = diastolic pressure:

$$MAP = \frac{(D \times 2) + S}{3}$$

(M-S)

▓ *Hemodilution of pregnancy* is the increase in blood volume that occurs during pregnancy. The increased volume consists of plasma and causes an imbalance between the ratio of red blood cells to plasma and a resultant decrease in hematocrit.   **(MAT)**

▓ Mean arterial pressure of greater than 100 mm Hg after 20 weeks of pregnancy is considered hypertension.   **(MAT)**

Symptoms of supine hypotension syndrome are dizziness, light-headedness, nausea, and vomiting.   (M-S)

The treatment for supine hypotension syndrome (a condition that sometimes occurs in pregnancy) is to have the patient lie on her left side.
                                                                        (MAT)

A contributing factor in dependent edema in the pregnant patient is the increase of femoral venous pressure from 10 mm Hg (normal) to 18 mm Hg (high).   (MAT)

Hyperpigmentation of the pregnant patient's face, formerly called *chloasma* and now referred to as *melasma*, fades after delivery.   (MAT)

The hormone relaxin, which is secreted first by the corpus luteum and later by the placenta, relaxes the connective tissue and cartilage of the symphysis pubis and the sacroiliac joint to facilitate passage of the fetus during delivery.   (MAT)

Progesterone maintains the integrity of the pregnancy by inhibiting uterine motility.   (MAT)

Ladin's sign, an early indication of pregnancy, causes softening of a spot on the anterior portion of the uterus, just above the uterocervical juncture.   (MAT)

During pregnancy, the abdominal line from the symphysis pubis to the umbilicus changes from linea alba to linea nigra.   (MAT)

In neonates, cold stress affects the circulatory, regulatory, and respiratory systems.   (MAT)

An immunocompromised patient is at risk for Kaposi's sarcoma. (M-S)

Obstetric data can be described by using the **F/TPAL** system:

F/T: Full-term delivery at 38 weeks or longer

P: Preterm delivery between 20 and 37 weeks

A: Abortion or loss of fetus before 20 weeks

L: Number of children living (if a child has died, further explanation is needed to clarify the discrepancy in numbers).   (MAT)

Parity doesn't refer to the number of infants delivered, only the number of deliveries.   (MAT)

- Women who are carrying more than one fetus should be encouraged to gain 35 to 45 lb (15.5 to 20.5 kg) during pregnancy.   (MAT)

- The recommended amount of iron supplement for the pregnant patient is 30 to 60 mg daily.   (MAT)

- Drinking six alcoholic beverages a day or a single episode of binge drinking in the first trimester can cause fetal alcohol syndrome.   (MAT)

- Chorionic villus sampling is performed at 8 to 12 weeks of pregnancy for early identification of genetic defects.   (MAT)

- In percutaneous umbilical blood sampling, a blood sample is obtained from the umbilical cord to detect anemia, genetic defects, and blood incompatibility as well as to assess the need for blood transfusions. (MAT)

- The period between contractions is referred to as the *interval,* or *resting phase.* During this phase, the uterus and placenta fill with blood and allow for the exchange of oxygen, carbon dioxide, and nutrients.   (MAT)

- In a patient who has hypertonic contractions, the uterus doesn't have an opportunity to relax and there is no interval between contractions. As a result, the fetus may experience hypoxia or rapid delivery may occur.   (MAT)

- Two qualities of the myometrium are elasticity, which allows it to stretch yet maintain its tone, and contractility, which allows it to shorten and lengthen in a synchronized pattern.   (MAT)

- During crowning, the presenting part of the fetus remains visible during the interval between contractions.   (MAT)

- *Uterine atony* is failure of the uterus to remain firmly contracted. (MAT)

- The major cause of uterine atony is a full bladder.   (MAT)

- If the mother wishes to breast-feed, the neonate should be nursed as soon as possible after delivery.   (MAT)

- A smacking sound, milk dripping from the side of the mouth, and sucking noises all indicate improper placement of the infant's mouth over the nipple.   (MAT)

- Before feeding is initiated, an infant should be burped to expel air from the stomach.   (MAT)

Most authorities strongly encourage the continuation of breast-feeding on both the affected and the unaffected breast of patients with mastitis. **(MAT)**

Expiratory grunting is an abnormal breath sound that's heard as an infant attempts to breathe out against a closed glottis. **(PED)**

On an infant, the abdomen is the ideal place to check skin turgor. **(PED)**

In infants, normal urine output is 1 to 3 ml/kg of body weight per hour. **(PED)**

Doll's eye movement is the normal lag between head movement and eye movement. **(M-S)**

Neonates are nearsighted and focus on items that are held 10″ to 12″ (25 to 30.5 cm) away. **(MAT)**

In a neonate, low-set ears are associated with chromosomal abnormalities such as Down syndrome. **(MAT)**

Meconium is usually passed in the first 24 hours; however, passage may take up to 72 hours. **(MAT)**

Breast-fed infants tend to pass feces that are looser and pastier than those of bottle-fed babies. **(PED)**

Boys who are born with hypospadias shouldn't be circumcised at birth because the foreskin may be needed for constructive surgery. **(MAT)**

Circumcision performed by a rabbi is called a *bris*. **(PED)**

The most desirable diet for an infant up to age 6 months is breast milk. **(PED)**

A bottle-fed infant is ready for the addition of solids to his diet when he meets these criteria: He has doubled his birth weight. He demands 8 to 10 feedings in a 24-hour period. He drinks more than 1 qt of formula a day. He always seems hungry. **(PED)**

Solids are introduced to the infant in the following order: rice cereal, fruits, oatmeal, vegetables, and meat. **(PED)**

In the neonate, the normal blood glucose level is 45 to 90 mg/dl. **(MAT)**

■ Hepatitis B vaccine is usually given within 48 hours of birth. **(MAT)**

■ Hepatitis B immune globulin is usually given within 12 hours of birth. **(MAT)**

■ HELLP (hemolysis, elevated liver enzymes, and low platelets) syndrome is an unusual variation of pregnancy-induced hypertension. **(MAT)**

■ Maternal serum alpha-fetoprotein is detectable at 7 weeks of gestation and peaks in the third trimester. High levels detected between the 16th and 18th weeks are associated with neural tube defects. Low levels are associated with Down syndrome. **(MAT)**

■ An arrest of descent occurs when the fetus doesn't descend through the pelvic cavity during labor. It's commonly associated with cephalopelvic disproportion, and cesarean delivery may be required. **(MAT)**

■ A late sign of preeclampsia is epigastric pain as a result of severe liver edema. **(MAT)**

■ In the patient with preeclampsia, blood pressure returns to normal during the puerperal period. **(MAT)**

■ Third spacing of fluid occurs when fluid shifts from the intravascular space to the interstitial space and remains there. **(M-S)**

■ *Chronic pain* is any pain that lasts longer than 6 months. *Acute pain* lasts less than 6 months. **(M-S)**

■ *Double-bind communication* occurs when the verbal message contradicts the nonverbal message and the receiver is unsure of which message to respond to. **(FND)**

■ A nonjudgmental attitude displayed by a nurse shows that she neither approves nor disapproves of the patient. **(FND)**

■ In a psychiatric setting, the patient should be able to predict the nurse's behavior and expect consistent positive attitudes and approaches. **(PSY)**

■ When establishing a schedule for a one-to-one interaction with a patient, the nurse should state how long the conversation will last and then adhere to the time limit. **(PSY)**

■ Target symptoms are those that the patient finds most distressing. **(FND)**

The mechanism of action of a phenothiazine derivative is to block dopamine receptors in the brain.   (M-S)

Thought broadcasting is a type of delusion in which the person believes that his thoughts are being broadcast for the world to hear.   (PSY)

A patient should be advised to take aspirin on an empty stomach, with a full glass of water, and should avoid acidic foods such as coffee, citrus fruits, and cola.   (FND)

Patients shouldn't take bisacodyl, antacids, and dairy products all at the same time.   (M-S)

Advise the patient who is taking digoxin to avoid foods that are high in fiber, such as bran cereal and prunes.   (M-S)

A patient who is taking diuretics should avoid foods that contain monosodium glutamate because it can cause tightening of the chest and flushing of the face.   (M-S)

Furosemide (Lasix) should be taken 1 hour before meals.   (M-S)

A patient who is taking griseofulvin (Grisovin FP) should maintain a high-fat diet, which enhances the secretion of bile.   (M-S)

Patients should take oral iron products with citrus drinks to enhance absorption.   (M-S)

Isoniazid should be taken on an empty stomach, with a full glass of water.   (M-S)

Foods that are high in protein decrease the absorption of levodopa.   (M-S)

Lithium should be taken with food. A patient who is taking lithium shouldn't restrict his sodium intake.   (PSY)

A patient who is taking lithium should stop taking the drug and call his physician if he experiences vomiting, drowsiness, or muscle weakness.   (PSY)

A patient who is taking tetracycline shouldn't take iron supplements or antacids.   (M-S)

A patient who is taking warfarin (Coumadin) should avoid foods that are high in vitamin K, such as liver and green leafy vegetables.   (M-S)

■ The patient who is taking a monoamine oxidase inhibitor for depression can include cottage cheese, cream cheese, yogurt, and sour cream in his diet.   (PSY)

■ The normal value for cholesterol is less than 200 mg/dl. The normal value for low-density lipoproteins is 60 to 180 mg/dl; for high-density lipoproteins, it's 30 to 80 mg/dl.   (M-S)

■ The normal cardiac output for an adult who weighs 155 lb (70.3 kg) is 5 to 6 L/minute.   (M-S)

■ A pulmonary artery pressure catheter (Swan-Ganz) measures the pressure in the cardiac chambers.   (M-S)

■ Severe chest pain that's aggravated by breathing and is described as "sharp," "stabbing," or "knifelike" is consistent with pericarditis. (M-S)

■ *Water-hammer pulse* is a pulse that's loud and bounding and rises and falls rapidly. It can be caused by emotional excitement or aortic insufficiency.   (M-S)

■ Pathologic splitting of S_2 is normally heard between inspiration and expiration. It occurs in right bundle-branch block.   (M-S)

■ Pink, frothy sputum is associated with pulmonary edema. Frank hemoptysis may be associated with pulmonary embolism.   (M-S)

■ An aortic aneurysm can be heard just over the umbilical area and can be detected as an abdominal pulsation (bruit).   (M-S)

■ Heart murmurs are graded according to the following system: grade 1 is faint and is heard after the examiner "tunes in"; grade 2 is heard immediately; grade 3 is moderately loud; grade 4 is loud; grade 5 is very loud, but is heard only with a stethoscope; and grade 6 is very loud and is heard without a stethoscope.   (M-S)

■ Clot formation during cardiac catheterization is minimized by the administration of 4,000 to 5,000 units of heparin.   (M-S)

■ Most complications that arise from cardiac catheterization are associated with the puncture site.   (M-S)

■ Allergic symptoms associated with iodine-based contrast media used in cardiac catheterization include urticaria, nausea and vomiting, and flushing.   (M-S)

■ To ensure that blood flow hasn't been compromised, the nurse should mark the peripheral pulses distal to the cutdown site to aid in locating the pulses after the procedure.   (M-S)

■ The extremity used for the cutdown site should remain straight for 4 to 6 hours. If an antecubital vessel was used, an armboard is needed. If a femoral artery was used, the patient should remain on bed rest for 6 to 12 hours.   (M-S)

■ If a patient experiences numbness or tingling in the extremity after a cutdown, the physician should be notified immediately.   (M-S)

■ After cardiac catheterization, fluid intake should be encouraged to aid in flushing the contrast medium through the kidneys.   (M-S)

■ In a patient who is undergoing pulmonary artery catheterization, risks include pulmonary artery infarction, pulmonary embolism, injury to the heart valves, and injury to the myocardium.   (M-S)

■ Pulmonary artery wedge pressure is a direct indicator of left ventricular pressure.   (M-S)

■ Pulmonary artery wedge pressure greater than 18 to 20 mm Hg indicates increased left ventricular pressure, as seen in left-sided heart failure.
    (M-S)

■ When measuring pulmonary artery wedge pressure, the nurse should place the patient in a supine position, with the head of the bed elevated no more than 25 degrees.   (M-S)

■ Pulmonary artery pressure, which indicates right and left ventricular pressure, is taken with the balloon deflated.   (M-S)

■ Pulmonary artery systolic pressure is the peak pressure generated by the right ventricle. Pulmonary artery diastolic pressure is the lowest pressure in the pulmonary artery.   (M-S)

■ Normal adult pulmonary artery systolic pressure is 15 to 25 mm Hg.
    (M-S)

■ Normal adult pulmonary artery diastolic pressure is 8 to 12 mm Hg.
    (M-S)

■ The normal oxygen saturation of venous blood is 75%.   (M-S)

▓ *Central venous pressure* is the amount of pressure in the superior vena cava and the right atrium. **(M-S)**

▓ Normal adult central venous pressure is 2 to 8 mm Hg, or 3 to 10 cm H_2O. **(M-S)**

▓ A decrease in central venous pressure indicates a fall in circulating fluid volume, as seen in shock. **(M-S)**

▓ An increase in central venous pressure is associated with an increase in circulating volume, as seen in renal failure. **(M-S)**

▓ In a patient who is on a ventilator, central venous pressure should be taken at the end of the expiratory cycle. **(M-S)**

▓ To ensure an accurate baseline central venous pressure reading, the zero point of the transducer must be at the level of the right atrium. **(M-S)**

▓ A blood pressure reading obtained through intra-arterial pressure monitoring may be 10 mm Hg higher than one obtained with a blood pressure cuff. **(M-S)**

▓ In Mönckeberg's sclerosis, calcium deposits form in the medial layer of the arterial walls. **(M-S)**

▓ The symptoms associated with coronary artery disease usually don't appear until plaque has narrowed the vessels by at least 75%. **(M-S)**

▓ Symptoms of coronary artery disease appear only when there is an imbalance between the demand for oxygenated blood and its availability. **(M-S)**

▓ Percutaneous transluminal coronary angioplasty is an invasive procedure in which a balloon-tipped catheter is inserted into a blocked artery. When the balloon is inflated, it opens the artery by compressing plaque against the artery's intimal layer. **(M-S)**

▓ Before percutaneous transluminal coronary angioplasty is performed, an anticoagulant (such as aspirin) is usually administered to the patient. During the procedure, the patient is given heparin, a calcium agonist, or nitroglycerin to reduce the risk of coronary artery spasms. **(M-S)**

▓ During coronary artery bypass graft surgery, a blocked coronary artery is bypassed by using the saphenous vein from the patient's thigh or lower leg. **(M-S)**

- When a vein is used to bypass an artery, the vein is reversed so that the valves don't interfere with blood flow.   (M-S)

- During a coronary artery bypass graft procedure, the patient's heart is stopped to allow the surgeon to sew the new vessel in place. Blood flow to the body is maintained with a cardiopulmonary bypass.   (M-S)

- During an anginal attack, the cells of the heart convert to anaerobic metabolism, which produces lactic acid as a waste product. As the level of lactic acid increases, pain develops.   (M-S)

- Pain that's described as "sharp" or "knifelike" is not consistent with angina pectoris.   (M-S)

- Anginal pain typically lasts for 5 minutes; however, attacks associated with a heavy meal or extreme emotional distress may last 15 to 20 minutes.   (M-S)

- A pattern of "exertion-pain-rest-relief" is consistent with stable angina.   (M-S)

- Unlike stable angina, unstable angina can occur without exertion and is considered a precursor to a myocardial infarction.   (M-S)

- A patient who is scheduled for a stress electrocardiogram should notify the staff if he has taken nitrates. If he has, the test must be rescheduled.   (M-S)

- Exercise equipment, such as a treadmill or an exercise bike, is used for a stress electrocardiogram. Activity is increased until the patient reaches 85% of his maximum heart rate.   (M-S)

- In patients who take nitroglycerin for a long time, tolerance often develops and reduces the effectiveness of nitrates. A 12-hour drug-free period is usually maintained at night.   (M-S)

- Beta-adrenergic blockers, such as propranolol (Inderal), reduce the workload on the heart, thereby decreasing oxygen demand. They also slow the heart rate.   (M-S)

- Calcium channel blockers include nifedipine (Procardia), which is used to treat angina; verapamil (Calan, Isoptin), which is used primarily as an antiarrhythmic; and diltiazem (Cardizem), which combines the effects of nifedipine and verapamil without the adverse effects.   (M-S)

▦ A patient who has anginal pain that radiates or worsens and doesn't subside should be evaluated at an emergency medical facility.   (M-S)

▦ Cardiac cells can withstand 20 minutes of ischemia before cell death occurs.   (M-S)

▦ During a myocardial infarction, the most common site of injury is the anterior wall of the left ventricle, near the apex.   (M-S)

▦ After a myocardial infarction, the infarcted tissue causes significant Q-wave changes on an electrocardiogram. These changes remain evident even after the myocardium heals.   (M-S)

▦ The level of CK-MB, an isoenzyme specific to the heart, increases 4 to 6 hours after a myocardial infarction and peaks at 12 to 18 hours. It returns to normal in 3 to 4 days.   (M-S)

▦ Patients who survive a myocardial infarction and have no other cardiovascular pathology usually require 6 to 12 weeks for a full recovery.   (M-S)

▦ After a myocardial infarction, the patient is at greatest risk for sudden death during the first 24 hours.   (M-S)

▦ After a myocardial infarction, the first 6 hours is the crucial period for salvaging the myocardium.   (M-S)

▦ After a myocardial infarction, if the patient consistently has more than three premature ventricular contractions per minute, the physician should be notified.   (M-S)

▦ After a myocardial infarction, increasing vascular resistance through the use of vasopressors, such as dopamine and levarterenol, can raise blood pressure.   (M-S)

▦ Clinical manifestations of heart failure include distended neck veins, weight gain, orthopnea, crackles, and enlarged liver.   (M-S)

▦ Risk factors associated with embolism are increased blood viscosity, decreased circulation, prolonged bed rest, and increased blood coagulability.   (M-S)

▦ Antiembolism stockings should be worn around the clock, but should be removed twice a day for 30 minutes so that skin care can be performed.   (M-S)

Before the nurse puts antiembolism stockings back on the patient, the patient should lie with his feet elevated 6″ (15.2 cm) for 20 minutes. **(M-S)**

Dressler's syndrome is known as *late pericarditis* because it occurs approximately 6 weeks to 6 months after a myocardial infarction. It causes pericardial pain and a fever that lasts longer than 1 week. **(M-S)**

In phase I after a myocardial infarction, for the first 24 hours, the patient is kept on a clear liquid diet and bed rest with the use of a bedside commode. **(M-S)**

In phase I after a myocardial infarction, on the second day, the patient gets out of bed and spends 15 to 20 minutes in a chair. The number of times that the patient goes to the chair and the length of time he spends in the chair are increased depending on his endurance. In phase II, the length of time that the patient spends out of bed and the distance to the chair are increased. **(M-S)**

After transfer from the cardiac care unit, the post-myocardial infarction patient is allowed to walk the halls as his endurance increases. **(M-S)**

Sexual intercourse with a known partner usually can be resumed 4 to 8 weeks after a myocardial infarction. **(M-S)**

A patient under cardiac care should avoid drinking alcoholic beverages or eating before engaging in sexual intercourse. **(M-S)**

The ambulation goal for a post-myocardial infarction patient is 2 miles in 60 minutes. **(M-S)**

A post-myocardial infarction patient who doesn't have a strenuous job may be able to return to work full-time in 8 or 9 weeks. **(M-S)**

Stroke volume is the amount of blood ejected from the heart with each heartbeat. **(M-S)**

Afterload is the force that the ventricle must exert during systole to eject the stroke volume. **(M-S)**

The three-point position (with the patient upright and leaning forward, with the hands on the knees) is characteristic of orthopnea, as seen in left-sided heart failure. **(M-S)**

- Paroxysmal nocturnal dyspnea indicates a severe form of pulmonary congestion in which the patient awakens in the middle of the night with a feeling of being suffocated. **(M-S)**

- Clinical manifestations of pulmonary edema include breathlessness, nasal flaring, use of accessory muscles to breath, and frothy sputum. **(M-S)**

- A late sign of heart failure is decreased cardiac output that causes decreased blood flow to the kidneys and results in oliguria. **(M-S)**

- A late sign of heart failure is anasarca (generalized edema). **(M-S)**

- Dependent edema is an early sign of right-sided heart failure. It's seen in the legs, where increased capillary hydrostatic pressure overwhelms plasma protein, causing a shift of fluid from the capillary beds to the interstitial spaces. **(M-S)**

- Dependent edema, which is most noticeable at the end of the day, usually starts in the feet and ankles and continues upward. **(M-S)**

- For the recumbent patient, edema is usually seen in the presacral area. **(M-S)**

- Signs of urinary tract infection include frequency, urgency, and dysuria. **(M-S)**

- In tertiary-intention healing, wound closure is delayed because of infection or edema. **(M-S)**

- A patient who has had supratentorial surgery should have the head of the bed elevated 30 degrees. **(M-S)**

- An acid-ash diet acidifies urine. **(M-S)**

- Vitamin C and cranberry juice acidify urine. **(M-S)**

- A patient who takes probenecid (ColBenemid) for gout should be instructed to take the drug with food. **(M-S)**

- If wound dehiscence is suspected, the nurse should instruct the patient to lie down and should examine the wound and monitor the vital signs. Abnormal findings should be reported to the physician. **(M-S)**

- Zoster immune globulin is administered to stimulate immunity to varicella. **(M-S)**

The most common symptoms associated with compartmental syndrome are pain that's not relieved by analgesics, loss of movement, loss of sensation, pain with passive movement, and lack of pulse.   **(M-S)**

To help relieve muscle spasms in a patient who has multiple sclerosis, the nurse should administer baclofen (Lioresal) as ordered; give the patient a warm, soothing bath; and teach the patient progressive relaxation techniques.   **(M-S)**

A patient who has a cervical injury and impairment at C5 should be able to lift his shoulders and elbows partially, but has no sensation below the clavicle.   **(M-S)**

A patient who has cervical injury and impairment at C6 should be able to lift his shoulders, elbows, and wrists partially, but has no sensation below the clavicle, except a small amount in the arms and thumb.

(M-S)

A patient who has cervical injury and impairment at C7 should be able to lift his shoulders, elbows, wrists, and hands partially, but has no sensation below the midchest.   **(M-S)**

Injuries to the spinal cord at C3 and above may be fatal as a result of loss of innervation to the diaphragm and intercostal muscles.   **(M-S)**

For every patient problem, there is a nursing diagnosis; for every nursing diagnosis, there is a goal; and for every goal, there are interventions designed to make the goal a reality. The keys to answering examination questions correctly are identifying the problem presented, formulating a goal for the problem, and selecting the intervention from the choices provided that will enable the patient to reach that goal.   **(FND)**

Signs of meningeal irritation seen in meningitis include nuchal rigidity, a positive Brudzinski's sign, and a positive Kernig's sign.   **(M-S)**

Laboratory values that show pneumomeningitis include an elevated cerebrospinal fluid (CSF) protein level (more than 100 mg/dl), a decreased CSF glucose level (40 mg/dl), and an increased white blood cell count.

(M-S)

To promote rest in a very young child in a hospital setting, the first nursing action is to decrease environmental stimulation.   **(PED)**

To promote sleep in a very young child in a hospital setting, the nurse should ask the parents about the child's sleep rituals.   **(PED)**

▓ Before undergoing magnetic resonance imaging, the patient should remove all objects containing metal, such as watches, underwire bras, and jewelry.   **(M-S)**

▓ Usually food and medicine aren't restricted before magnetic resonance imaging.   **(M-S)**

▓ Patients who are undergoing magnetic resonance imaging should know that they can ask questions during the procedure; however, they may be asked to lie still at certain times.   **(M-S)**

▓ If a contrast medium is used during magnetic resonance imaging, the patient may experience diuresis as the medium is flushed from the body.
                                                                                  (M-S)

▓ The Tzanck test is used to confirm herpes genitalis.   **(M-S)**

▓ Hepatitis C is spread primarily through blood (for example, during transfusion or in people who work with blood products), personal contact and, possibly, the fecal-oral route.   **(M-S)**

▓ The best method for soaking an open, infected, draining wound is to use a hot-moist dressing.   **(M-S)**

▓ Sputum culture is the confirmation test for tuberculosis.   **(M-S)**

▓ Dexamethasone (Decadron) is a steroidal anti-inflammatory that's used to treat adrenal insufficiency.   **(M-S)**

▓ Signs of increased intracranial pressure include alteration in level of consciousness, restlessness, irritability, and pupillary changes.   **(M-S)**

▓ The patient who has a lower limb amputation should be instructed to assume a prone position at least twice a day.   **(M-S)**

▓ During the first 24 hours after amputation, the residual limb is elevated on a pillow. After that time, the limb is placed flat to reduce the risk of hip flexion contractures.   **(M-S)**

▓ A tourniquet should be in full view at the bedside of the patient who has an amputation.   **(M-S)**

▓ An emergency tracheostomy set should be kept at the bedside of a patient who is suspected of having epiglottitis.   **(M-S)**

Rocky Mountain spotted fever is spread through the bite of a tick harboring the *Rickettsia* organism.   (M-S)

In reporting suspected cases of child abuse to the appropriate authorities, the key word to use is "suspected."   (PED)

A patient who has acquired immunodeficiency syndrome shouldn't share razors or toothbrushes with others, but there are no special precautions for dinnerware or laundry services.   (M-S)

Because antifungal creams may stain clothing, patients who use them should use sanitary napkins.   (M-S)

An antifungal cream should be inserted high in the vagina at bedtime.
                                                                       (M-S)

A patient who is having a seizure usually requires protection from the environment only; however, anyone who needs airway management should be turned on his side.   (M-S)

Status epilepticus is treated with I.V. diphenylhydantoin.   (M-S)

A *xenograft* is a skin graft from an animal.   (M-S)

Fidelity means loyalty and can be shown as a commitment to the profession of nursing and to the patient.   (FND)

Administering an I.M. injection against the patient's will and without legal authority is battery.   (FND)

An example of a third-party payer is an insurance company.   (FND)

The formula for calculating the drops per minute for an I.V. infusion is as follows:

$$\frac{(\text{volume to be infused} \times \text{drip factor})}{\text{time in minutes}} = \text{drops/minute}$$
                                                                       (FND)

On-call medication should be given within 5 minutes of the call. (FND)

Usually, the best method to determine a patient's cultural or spiritual needs is to ask him.   (FND)

An incident report or unusual occurrence report isn't part of a patient's record, but is an in-house document that's used for the purpose of correcting the problem.   (FND)

▨ Critical pathways are a multidisciplinary guideline for patient care.

(FND)

▨ The antidote for magnesium sulfate is calcium gluconate 10%.   (M-S)

▨ Allergic reactions to a blood transfusion are flushing, wheezing, urticaria, and rash.   (M-S)

▨ A child who has asthma can promote expansion of the lungs by blowing a pinwheel.   (PED)

▨ A patient who has a history of basal cell carcinoma should avoid sun exposure.   (M-S)

▨ When potent, nitroglycerin causes a slight stinging sensation under the tongue.   (M-S)

▨ To obtain an estriol level, urine is collected for 24 hours.   (MAT)

▨ An estriol level is used to assess fetal well-being and maternal renal functioning as well as to monitor a pregnancy that's complicated by diabetes.

(MAT)

▨ A patient who appears to be "fighting the ventilator" is holding his breath or breathing out on an inspiratory cycle.   (M-S)

▨ An antineoplastic drug that's used to treat breast cancer is tamoxifen (Nolvadex).   (M-S)

▨ Adverse effects of vincristine (Oncovin) are alopecia, nausea, and vomiting.   (M-S)

▨ A pregnant patient with vaginal bleeding shouldn't have a pelvic examination.   (MAT)

▨ Increased urine output is an indication that a hypertensive crisis is normalizing.   (M-S)

▨ If a patient who is receiving I.V. chemotherapy has pain at the insertion site, the nurse should stop the I.V. infusion immediately.   (M-S)

▨ *Extravasation* is leakage of fluid into surrounding tissue from a vein that's being used for I.V. therapy.   (M-S)

▨ Clinical signs of prostate cancer are dribbling, hesitancy, and decreased urinary force.   (M-S)

■ Cardiac glycosides increase cardiac contractility.   **(M-S)**

■ Adverse effects of cardiac glycosides include headache, hypotension, nausea and vomiting, and yellow-green halos around lights.   **(M-S)**

■ A T tube should be clamped during patient meals to aid in fat digestion.   **(M-S)**

■ A T tube usually remains in place for 10 days.   **(M-S)**

■ During a vertigo attack, a patient who has Ménière's disease should be instructed to lie down on his side with his eyes closed.   **(M-S)**

■ When prioritizing nursing diagnoses, the following hierarchy should be used: Problems associated with the airway, those concerning breathing, and those related to circulation.   **(FND)**

■ The two nursing diagnoses that have the highest priority that the nurse can assign are *Ineffective airway clearance* and *Ineffective breathing pattern*.   **(FND)**

■ When maintaining a Jackson-Pratt drainage system, the nurse should squeeze the reservoir and expel the air before recapping the system.   **(M-S)**

■ *Sensory overload* is a state in which sensory stimulation exceeds the individual's capacity to tolerate or process it.   **(PSY)**

■ Symptoms of sensory overload include a feeling of distress and hyperarousal with impaired thinking and concentration.   **(PSY)**

■ In sensory deprivation, overall sensory input is decreased.   **(PSY)**

■ A sign of sensory deprivation is a decrease in stimulation from the environment or from within oneself, such as daydreaming, inactivity, sleeping excessively, and reminiscing.   **(PSY)**

■ A subjective sign that a sitz bath has been effective is the patient's expression of decreased pain or discomfort.   **(FND)**

■ For the nursing diagnosis *Deficient diversional activity* to be valid, the patient must state that he's "bored," that he has "nothing to do," or words to that effect.   **(FND)**

■ The most appropriate nursing diagnosis for an individual who doesn't speak English is *Impaired verbal communication related to inability to speak dominant language (English)*.   **(FND)**

■ The family of a patient who has been diagnosed as hearing impaired should be instructed to face the individual when they speak to him.
(FND)

■ The most common symptom associated with sleep apnea is snoring.
(M-S)

■ Before instilling medication into the ear of a patient who is up to age 3, the nurse should pull the pinna down and back to straighten the eustachian tube.   **(FND)**

■ To prevent injury to the cornea when administering eyedrops, the nurse should waste the first drop and instill the drug in the lower conjunctival sac.   **(FND)**

■ After administering eye ointment, the nurse should twist the medication tube to detach the ointment.   **(FND)**

■ Histamine is released during an inflammatory response.   **(M-S)**

■ When dealing with a patient who has a severe speech impediment, the nurse should minimize background noise and avoid interrupting the patient.   **(M-S)**

■ Fever and night sweats, hallmark signs of tuberculosis, may not be present in elderly patients who have the disease.   **(M-S)**

■ A suitable dressing for wound debridement is wet-to-dry.   **(M-S)**

■ Drinking warm milk at bedtime aids sleeping because of the natural sedative effect of the amino acid tryptophan.   **(M-S)**

■ The three stages of general adaptation syndrome are alarm, resistance, and exhaustion.   **(PSY)**

■ The initial step in promoting sleep in a hospitalized patient is to minimize environmental stimulation.   **(M-S)**

Before moving a patient, the nurse should assess how much exertion the patient is permitted, the patient's physical ability, and his ability to understand instruction as well as her own strength and ability to move the patient.   **(M-S)**

A patient who is in a restraint should be checked every 30 minutes and the restraint loosened every 2 hours to permit range of motion exercises for the extremities.   **(M-S)**

Antibiotics that are given four times a day should be given at 6 a.m., 12 p.m., 6 p.m., and 12 a.m. to minimize disruption of sleep.   **(M-S)**

When the nurse removes gloves and a mask, she should remove the gloves first. They are soiled and are likely to contain pathogens.   **(FND)**

Sundowner syndrome is seen in patients who become more confused toward the evening. To counter this tendency, the nurse should turn a light on.   **(M-S)**

Crutches should be placed 6" (15.2 cm) in front of the patient and 6" to the side to form a tripod arrangement.   **(FND)**

For the patient who has somnambulism, the primary goal is to prevent injury by providing a safe environment.   **(M-S)**

Naloxone (Narcan) should be kept at the bedside of the patient who is receiving patient-controlled analgesia.   **(M-S)**

Listening is the most effective communication technique.   **(FND)**

Hypnotic drugs decrease rapid eye movement sleep, but increase the overall amount of sleep.   **(M-S)**

Before teaching any procedure to a patient, the nurse must assess the patient's current knowledge and willingness to learn.   **(FND)**

A sudden wave of overwhelming sleepiness is a symptom of narcolepsy.
                                                                                                                  (M-S)

Process recording is a method of evaluating one's communication effectiveness.   **(FND)**

When feeding an elderly patient, the nurse should limit high-carbohydrate foods because of the risk of glucose intolerance.   **(FND)**

■ When feeding an elderly patient, essential foods should be given first. (FND)

■ Passive range of motion maintains joint mobility. Resistive exercises increase muscle mass. (FND)

■ Isometric exercises are performed on an extremity that's in a cast. (FND)

■ A diabetic patient should be instructed to buy shoes in the afternoon because feet are usually largest at that time of day. (M-S)

■ A maladaptive response to stress is drinking alcohol or smoking excessively. (PSY)

■ A back rub is an example of the gate-control theory of pain. (FND)

■ Anything that's located below the waist is considered unsterile; a sterile field becomes unsterile when it comes in contact with any unsterile item; a sterile field must be monitored continuously; and a border of 1″ (2.5 cm) around a sterile field is considered unsterile. (FND)

■ A "shift to the left" is evident when the number of immature cells (bands) in the blood increases to fight an infection. (FND)

■ A "shift to the right" is evident when the number of mature cells in the blood increases, as seen in advanced liver disease and pernicious anemia. (FND)

■ If surgery is scheduled late in the afternoon, the surgeon may approve a light breakfast. (M-S)

■ A hearing aid is usually left in place during surgery to permit communication with the patient. The operating room team should be notified of its presence. (M-S)

■ Before administering preoperative medication, the nurse should ensure that an informed consent form has been signed and attached to the patient's record. (FND)

■ The nurse should monitor the patient for central nervous system depression for 24 hours after the administration of nitrous oxide. (M-S)

■ In the postanesthesia care unit, the proper position of an adult is with the head to the side and the chin extended upward. The Sims' position also can be used unless contraindicated. (M-S)

▓ After a patient is admitted to the postanesthesia care unit, the first action is to assess the patency of the airway. (M-S)

▓ If a patient is admitted to the postanesthesia care unit without the pharyngeal reflex, he's positioned on his side. The nurse stays at the bedside until the gag reflex returns. (M-S)

▓ In the postanesthesia care unit, the patient's vital signs are taken every 15 minutes routinely, or more often if indicated, until the patient is stable. (M-S)

▓ In the postanesthesia care unit, the T tube should be unclamped and attached to a drainage system. (M-S)

▓ After the patient receives anesthesia, the nurse must observe him for a drop in blood pressure or evidence of labored breathing. (M-S)

▓ If a patient begins to go into shock during the postanesthesia assessment, the nurse should administer oxygen, place the patient in the Trendelenburg position, and increase the I.V. fluid rate according to the physician's order or the policy of the postanesthesia care unit. (M-S)

▓ Types of benign tumors include myxoma, fibroma, lipoma, osteoma, and chondroma. (M-S)

▓ Malignant tumors include sarcoma, basal cell carcinoma, fibrosarcoma, osteosarcoma, myxosarcoma, chondrosarcoma, and adenocarcinoma. (M-S)

▓ For a cancer patient, palliative surgery is performed to reduce pain, relieve airway obstruction, relieve GI obstruction, prevent hemorrhage, relieve pressure on the brain and spinal cord, drain abscesses, and remove or drain infected tumors. (M-S)

▓ A patient who is undergoing radiation implant therapy should be kept in a private room to reduce the risk of exposure to others, including nursing personnel. (M-S)

▓ A nurse should spend no more than 30 minutes per 8-hour shift providing care to a patient who has a radiation implant. (FND)

▓ A nurse shouldn't be assigned to care for more than one patient who has a radiation implant. (FND)

■ A masklike facial expression is a sign of myasthenia gravis and Parkinson's disease.   (M-S)

■ For the patient who abides by Jewish custom, milk and meat shouldn't be served at the same meal.   (FND)

■ Hyperalertness and the startle reflex are characteristics of posttraumatic stress disorder.   (PSY)

■ A treatment for a phobia is *desensitization,* a process in which the patient is slowly exposed to the feared stimuli.   (PSY)

■ Albumin is a colloid that aids in maintaining fluid within the vascular system. If albumin were filtered out through the kidneys and into the urine, edema would occur.   (M-S)

■ Edema caused by water and trauma doesn't cause pitting.   (M-S)

■ Dehydration is water loss only; fluid volume deficit includes all fluids in the body.   (M-S)

■ To maintain fluid balance, normal saline solution should be used when giving an enema to an infant.   (PED)

■ The primary action of an oil retention enema is to lubricate the colon. The secondary action is softening the feces.   (M-S)

■ In the early stages of pregnancy, the finding of glucose in the urine may be related to the increased shunting of glucose to the developing placenta, without a corresponding increase in the reabsorption capability of the kidneys.   (MAT)

■ A patient who uses a walker should be instructed to move the walker approximately 12″ (30.5 cm) to the front and then advance into the walker.   (M-S)

■ Bradykinesia is a sign of Parkinson's disease.   (M-S)

■ *Lordosis* is backward arching curvature of the spine.   (M-S)

■ *Kyphosis* is forward curvature of the spine.   (M-S)

■ A common symptom of acute lymphocytic leukemia in toddlers and preschoolers is leg pain.   (PED)

In a patient with anorexia nervosa, a positive response to therapy is sustained weight gain. (M-S)

The drug in dialysate is heparin. (M-S)

An *autograft* is a graft that's removed from one area of the body for transplantation to another. (M-S)

Signs of cervical cancer include midmenses bleeding and postcoital bleeding. (M-S)

After prostatectomy, a catheter is inserted to irrigate the bladder and keep urine straw-colored or light pink, to put direct pressure on the operative side, and to maintain a patent urethra. (M-S)

If a radiation implant becomes dislodged, but remains in the patient, the nurse should notify the physician. (M-S)

The best method to reduce the risk for atelectasis is to encourage the patient to walk. (M-S)

Atelectasis usually occurs 24 to 48 hours after surgery. (M-S)

Patients who are at the greatest risk for atelectasis are those who have had high abdominal surgery, such as cholecystectomy. (M-S)

A persistent decrease in oxygen to the kidneys causes erythropoiesis. (M-S)

Rhonchi and crackles indicate ineffective airway clearance. (M-S)

Wheezing indicates bronchospasms. (M-S)

Clinical signs and symptoms of hypoxemia are restlessness (usually the first sign), agitation, dyspnea, and disorientation. (M-S)

Common adverse effects of opioids are constipation and respiratory depression. (M-S)

Disuse osteoporosis is caused by demineralization of calcium as a result of prolonged bed rest. (M-S)

The best way to prevent disuse osteoporosis is to encourage the patient to walk. (M-S)

A patient who has premature rupture of the membranes is at significant risk for infection if labor doesn't begin within 24 hours. (MAT)

■ A cane should be carried on the unaffected side and advanced with the affected extremity. (M-S)

■ Steroids shouldn't be used in patients who have chickenpox or shingles because they may cause adverse effects. (M-S)

■ Seroconversion occurs approximately 3 to 6 months after exposure to human immunodeficiency virus. (M-S)

■ Therapy with the antiviral agent zidovudine is initiated when the CD4+ T-cell count is 500 cells/µl or less. (M-S)

■ In a light-skinned person, Kaposi's sarcoma causes a purplish discoloration of the skin. In a dark-skinned person, the discoloration is dark brown to black. (M-S)

■ After an esophageal balloon tamponade is in place, it should be inflated to 20 mm Hg. (M-S)

■ A patient who has Kaposi's sarcoma should avoid acidic or highly seasoned foods. (M-S)

■ The treatment for oral candidiasis is amphotericin B (Fungizone) or fluconazole (Diflucan). (M-S)

■ A sign of respiratory failure is vital capacity of less than 15 ml/kg and respiratory rate of greater than 30 breaths/minute or less than 8 breaths/minute. (M-S)

■ For left-sided cardiac catheterization, the catheter is threaded through the descending aorta, aortic arch, ascending aorta, aortic valve, and left ventricle. (M-S)

■ For right-sided cardiac catheterization, the catheter is threaded through the superior vena cava, right atrium, right ventricle, pulmonary artery, and pulmonary capillaries. (M-S)

■ Anemia can be divided into four groups according to its cause: blood loss, impaired production of red blood cells (RBCs), increased destruction of RBCs, and nutritional deficiencies. (M-S)

■ Aspirin, ibuprofen, phenobarbital, lithium, colchicine, lead, and chloramphenicol can cause aplastic anemia. (M-S)

After a patient undergoes bone marrow aspiration, the nurse should apply direct pressure to the site for 3 to 5 minutes to reduce the risk of bleeding.   (M-S)

Fresh frozen plasma is thawed to 98.6° F (37° C) before infusion. (M-S)

Signs of thrombocytopenia include petechiae, ecchymoses, hematuria, and gingival bleeding.   (M-S)

A patient who has thrombocytopenia should be taught to use a soft toothbrush and use an electric razor.   (M-S)

Signs of fluid overload include increased central venous pressure, increased pulse rate, distended jugular veins, and bounding pulse.   (M-S)

A patient who has leukopenia (or any other patient who is at an increased risk for infection) should avoid eating raw meat, fresh fruit, and fresh vegetables.   (M-S)

The peak age for the diagnosis of acute lymphocytic leukemia is ages 2 to 4.   (PED)

A patient who is undergoing therapy for acute lymphocytic leukemia should have his urine and feces checked for blood.   (PED)

To prevent a severe graft-versus-host reaction, which is most commonly seen in patients older than age 30, the donor marrow is treated with monoclonal antibodies before transplantation.   (M-S)

The four most common signs of hypoglycemia reported by patients are nervousness, mental disorientation, weakness, and perspiration.   (M-S)

Prolonged attacks of hypoglycemia in a diabetic patient can result in brain damage.   (M-S)

Whether the patient can perform a procedure (psychomotor domain of learning) is a better indicator of the effectiveness of patient teaching than whether the patient can simply state the steps involved in the procedure (cognitive domain of learning).   (FND)

Activities that increase intracranial pressure include coughing, sneezing, straining to pass feces, bending over, and blowing the nose.   (M-S)

Treatment for bleeding esophageal varices includes vasopressin, esophageal tamponade, iced saline lavage, and vitamin K.   (M-S)

▓ Hepatitis C (also known as blood-transfusion hepatitis) is a parenterally transmitted form of hepatitis that has a high incidence of carrier status. (M-S)

▓ The nurse should be concerned about fluid and electrolyte problems in the patient who has ascites, edema, decreased urine output, or low blood pressure. (M-S)

▓ The nurse should be concerned about GI bleeding, low blood pressure, and increased heart rate in a patient who is hemorrhaging. (M-S)

▓ The nurse should be concerned about generalized malaise, cloudy urine, purulent drainage, tachycardia, and increased temperature in a patient who has an infection. (M-S)

▓ In a patient who has edema or ascites, the serum electrolyte level should be monitored. The patient also should be weighed daily; have his abdominal girth measured with a centimeter tape at the same location, using the umbilicus as a checkpoint; have his intake and output measured; and have his blood pressure taken at least every 4 hours. (M-S)

▓ Endogenous sources of ammonia include azotemia, GI bleeding, catabolism, and constipation. (M-S)

▓ Exogenous sources of ammonia include protein, blood transfusion, and amino acids. (M-S)

▓ The following histologic grading system is used to classify cancers: grade 1, well-differentiated; grade 2, moderately well-differentiated; grade 3, poorly differentiated; and grade 4, very poorly differentiated. (M-S)

▓ The following grading system is used to classify tumors: T0, no evidence of a primary tumor; TIS, tumor in situ; and T1, T2, T3, and T4, according to the size and involvement of the tumor; the higher the number, the greater the involvement. (M-S)

▓ Symptoms of major depressive disorder include depressed mood, inability to experience pleasure, sleep disturbance, appetite changes, decreased libido, and feelings of worthlessness. (PSY)

- According to Erik Erikson, developmental stages are trust versus mistrust (birth to 18 months), autonomy versus shame and doubt (18 months to age 3), initiative versus guilt (ages 3 to 5), industry versus inferiority (ages 5 to 12), identity versus identity diffusion (ages 12 to 18), intimacy versus isolation (ages 18 to 25), generativity versus stagnation (ages 25 to 60), and ego integrity versus despair (older than age 60).   **(FND)**

- According to Sigmund Freud, the psychosexual stages of development are the oral stage (infancy, or birth to age 1), the anal stage (toddlerhood, or ages 1 to 3), the phallic stage (preschool age, or ages 3 to 6), the latency stage (school age, or ages 6 to 12), and the genital stage (adolescence and young adulthood, or ages 12 to 18).   **(PED)**

- Pheochromocytoma is a catecholamine-secreting neoplasm of the adrenal medulla. It causes excessive production of epinephrine and norepinephrine.   **(M-S)**

- Clinical manifestations of pheochromocytoma include visual disturbances, headaches, hypertension, and elevated serum glucose level.   **(M-S)**

- The patient shouldn't consume any caffeine-containing products, such as cola, coffee, or tea, for at least 8 hours before obtaining a 24-hour urine sample for vanillylmandelic acid.   **(M-S)**

- A patient who is taking ColBenemid (probenecid and colchicine) for gout should increase his fluid intake to 2,000 ml/day.   **(M-S)**

- A miotic such as pilocarpine is administered to a patient with glaucoma to increase the outflow of aqueous humor, which decreases intraocular tension.   **(M-S)**

- The drug that's most commonly used to treat streptococcal pharyngitis and rheumatic fever is penicillin.   **(M-S)**

- When communicating with a hearing impaired patient, the nurse should face him.   **(FND)**

- A patient with gout should avoid purine-containing foods, such as liver and other organ meats.   **(M-S)**

- A patient who undergoes magnetic resonance imaging lies on a flat platform that moves through a magnetic field.   **(M-S)**

- Infants of diabetic mothers are susceptible to macrosomia as a result of increased insulin production in the fetus. **(MAT)**

- Laboratory values in patients who have bacterial meningitis include increased white blood cell count, increased protein and lactic acid levels, and decreased glucose level. **(M-S)**

- To promote rest for a young child with meningitis, environmental stimulation should be decreased. **(PED)**

- Mannitol is a hypertonic osmotic diuretic that decreases intracranial pressure. **(M-S)**

- The best method to debride a wound is to use a wet-to-dry dressing and remove the dressing after it dries. **(M-S)**

- The greatest risk for respiratory complications occurs after chest wall injury, chest wall surgery, or upper abdominal surgery. **(M-S)**

- Secondary methods to prevent postoperative respiratory complications include having the patient use an incentive spirometer, turning the patient, advising the patient to cough and breathe deeply, and providing hydration. **(M-S)**

- The nurse shouldn't put anything (including a thermometer) in the mouth of a child who is suspected of having epiglottiditis. **(PED)**

- To prevent heat loss in the neonate, the nurse should bathe one part of his body at a time and keep the rest of the body covered. **(MAT)**

- A characteristic of allergic inspiratory and expiratory wheezing is a dry, hacking, nonproductive cough. **(M-S)**

- The incubation period for Rocky Mountain spotted fever is 7 to 14 days. **(M-S)**

- A spiral fracture of the humerus may indicate child abuse. **(PED)**

- Miconazole (Monistat) vaginal suppository should be administered with the patient lying flat. **(M-S)**

- The nurse should place the patient who is having a seizure on his side. **(M-S)**

- Signs of hip dislocation are one leg that's shorter than the other and one leg that's externally rotated. **(M-S)**

- Anticholinergic medication is administered before surgery to diminish secretion of saliva and gastric juices.   (M-S)

- Extrapyramidal syndrome in a patient with Parkinson's disease is usually caused by a deficiency of dopamine in the substantia nigra.   (M-S)

- In a burn patient, the order of concern is airway, circulation, pain, and infection.   (M-S)

- An appropriate nursing intervention for the spouse of a patient who has a serious incapacitating disease is to help him to mobilize a support system.   (FND)

- Hyperkalemia normally occurs during the hypovolemic phase in a patient who has a serious burn injury.   (M-S)

- Black feces in the burn patient are commonly related to Curling's ulcer.   (M-S)

- In a patient with burn injury, immediate care of a full-thickness skin graft includes covering the site with a bulky dressing.   (M-S)

- The donor site of a skin graft should be left exposed to the air.   (M-S)

- Leaking around a T tube should be reported immediately to the physician.   (M-S)

- A patient who has a cesarean delivery is at greater risk for infection than the patient who gives birth vaginally.   (MAT)

- A patient who has Ménière's disease should consume a low-sodium diet.   (M-S)

- In any postoperative patient, the priority of concern is airway, breathing, and circulation, followed by self-care deficits.   (M-S)

- The symptoms of myasthenia gravis are most likely related to nerve degeneration.   (M-S)

- Symptoms of septic shock include cold, clammy skin; hypotension; and decreased urine output.   (M-S)

- Ninety-five percent of women who have gonorrhea are asymptomatic.   (M-S)

- A sign of tinea capitis in the child is a scratch on the scalp.   (PED)

- Permethrin (Nix) shampoo for head lice is effective if there are no lice in the hair and no eggs (nits) fixed to hair shafts. (PED)

- An adverse sign in a patient who has a Steinmann's pin in the femur would be erythema, edema, and pain around the pin site. (M-S)

- Signs of chronic glaucoma include halos around lights, gradual loss of peripheral vision, and cloudy vision. (M-S)

- Signs of a detached retina include a sensation of a veil (or curtain) in the line of sight. (M-S)

- Toxic levels of streptomycin can cause hearing loss. (M-S)

- A long-term effect of rheumatic fever is mitral valve damage. (M-S)

- Laboratory values noted in rheumatic fever include an antistreptolysin-O titer, the presence of C-reactive protein, leukocytosis, and an increased erythrocyte sedimentation rate. (M-S)

- Crampy pain in the right lower quadrant of the abdomen is a consistent finding in Crohn's disease. (M-S)

- Crampy pain in the left lower quadrant of the abdomen is a consistent finding in diverticulitis. (M-S)

- In the icteric phase of hepatitis, urine is amber, feces are clay-colored, and the skin is yellow. (M-S)

- The occurrence of thrush in the neonate is probably caused by contact with the organism during delivery through the birth canal. (MAT)

- Signs of osteomyelitis include pathologic fractures, shortening or lengthening of the bone, and pain deep in the bone. (M-S)

- The laboratory test that would best reflect fluid loss because of a burn would be hematocrit. (M-S)

- Before administering digoxin to an infant, the nurse should take the apical pulse for 1 full minute. (PED)

- To determine how much urine is contained in a diaper, the nurse should weigh the wet diaper, subtract the weight of a dry diaper, and convert each gram to a milliliter (1 gram in weight = 1 milliliter in volume). (PED)

A patient who has acute pancreatitis should take nothing by mouth and undergo gastric suction to decompress the stomach. (M-S)

A mist tent is used to increase the hydration of secretions. (M-S)

A patient who is receiving levodopa should avoid foods that contain pyridoxine (vitamin B_6), such as beans, tuna, and beef liver, because this vitamin decreases the effectiveness of levodopa. (M-S)

A patient who has a transactional injury at C3 requires positive ventilation. (M-S)

The action of phenytoin (Dilantin) is potentiated when given with anticoagulants. (M-S)

Cerebral palsy is a nonprogressive disorder that persists throughout life. (M-S)

The nurse should keep the sac of meningomyelocele moist with normal saline solution. (MAT)

A consistent finding in a child with meningococcal meningitis is purpuric skin rash. (PED)

Treatment for a conscious toddler who has swallowed liquid drain cleaner is dilute vinegar solution. (PED)

A complication of ulcerative colitis is perforation. (M-S)

When a patient who has multiple sclerosis experiences diplopia, one eye should be patched. (M-S)

A danger sign after hip replacement is lack of reflexes in the affected extremity. (M-S)

A clinical manifestation of a ruptured lumbar disk includes pain that shoots down the leg and terminates in the popliteal space. (M-S)

When an infant is in a body cast, a diaper should be tucked into the perineal area to prevent urine from flowing back into the cast. (PED)

The most important nutritional need of the burn patient is I.V. fluid with electrolytes. (M-S)

After a child is given syrup of ipecac, he should bend over toward his knees. (PED)

The patient who has systemic lupus erythematosus should avoid sunshine, hair spray, hair coloring products, and dusting powder.   (M-S)

Poor hygiene is a contributing factor to the development of impetigo.   (PED)

The best position for a patient who has low back pain is sitting in a straight-backed chair.   (M-S)

Clinical signs of ulcerative colitis include bloody, purulent, mucoid, and watery feces.   (M-S)

A patient who has a protein systemic shunt must follow a lifelong protein-restricted diet.   (M-S)

A patient who has a hiatal hernia should maintain an upright position after eating.   (M-S)

A suction apparatus should be kept at the bedside of a patient who is at risk for status epilepticus.   (M-S)

The leading cause of death in the burn patient is respiratory compromise and infection.   (M-S)

Signs of scoliosis include limping walk, uneven hemline, and asymmetrical breasts.   (PED)

A measles-mumps-rubella vaccine shouldn't be given before age 12 months.   (PED)

An early sign of lead poisoning is drowsiness.   (PED)

Late signs of lead poisoning are seizures and irreversible brain damage.   (PED)

Pertussis vaccine shouldn't be given to a child whose blood test results show human immunodeficiency virus antibodies.   (PED)

In patients who have herpes zoster, the primary concern is pain management.   (M-S)

The treatment for Rocky Mountain spotted fever is tetracycline.   (M-S)

Strawberry tongue is a sign of scarlet fever.   (M-S)

Parents should inspect the bed linen of a child who has myringotomy tubes daily to ensure that the tubes haven't fallen out.   (PED)

If a patient has hemianopia, the nurse should place the call light, the meal tray, and other items in his field of vision.   (M-S)

A toddler in a crib should have a crib net.   (PED)

A child shouldn't be asked a "yes" or "no" question unless the nurse plans to follow the child's wishes.   (PED)

Bowlegs are a sign of Paget's disease.   (PED)

The best position for the patient after a craniotomy is semi-Fowler. (M-S)

The parent of a child who has a cast should watch for edema, which causes decreased capillary refill.   (PED)

Signs of renal trauma include flank pain, hematoma and, possibly, blood in the urine and decreased urine output.   (M-S)

Flank pain and hematoma in the back indicate renal hemorrhage in the trauma patient.   (M-S)

Natural diuretics include coffee, tea, and grapefruit juice.   (M-S)

Central venous pressure of 18 cm H_2O indicates hypervolemia.   (M-S)

Clinical signs of lithium toxicity are nausea, vomiting, and lethargy.
(PSY)

Salmonellosis can be acquired by eating contaminated meat such as chicken, or eggs.   (M-S)

Good sources of magnesium include fish, nuts, and grains.   (M-S)

Patients who have low blood urea nitrogen levels should be instructed to eat high-protein foods, such as fish and chicken.   (M-S)

The nurse should monitor a patient who has Guillain-Barré syndrome for respiratory compromise.   (M-S)

A heating pad may provide comfort to a patient who has pelvic inflammatory disease.   (M-S)

After supratentorial surgery, the patient should be placed in the semi-Fowler position.   (M-S)

■ To prevent deep vein thrombosis, the patient should exercise his legs at least every 2 hours, elevate the legs above the level of the heart while lying down, and ambulate with assistance.   (M-S)

■ After bronchoscopy, the patient's gag reflex should be checked.   (M-S)

■ In a patient with mononucleosis, abdominal pain and pain that radiates to the left shoulder may indicate a ruptured spleen.   (M-S)

■ For a skin graft to take, it must be autologous.   (M-S)

■ Untreated retinal detachment leads to blindness.   (M-S)

■ A patient who has fibrocystic breast disease should consume a diet that's low in caffeine and salt.   (M-S)

■ A foul odor at the pin site of a patient who is in skeletal traction indicates infection.   (M-S)

■ A muscle relaxant that's administered with oxygen may cause malignant hyperthermia and respiratory depression.   (M-S)

■ Pain that occurs on movement of the cervix, together with adnexal tenderness, suggests pelvic inflammatory disease.   (M-S)

■ Asking too many "why" questions yields scant information and may overwhelm a psychiatric patient and lead to stress and withdrawal.   (PSY)

■ If fundal height is at least 2 cm less than expected, the cause may be growth retardation, missed abortion, transverse lie, or false pregnancy.   (MAT)

■ In cyanotic congenital heart defects, unoxygenated blood is shunted from the right side of the heart to the left, where it flows through the left ventricle to all parts of the body, causing cyanosis.   (PED)

■ Fundal height that exceeds expectations by more than 2 cm may be caused by multiple gestation, polyhydramnios, uterine myomata, or a large baby.   (MAT)

■ Remote memory may be impaired in the late stages of dementia.   (PSY)

■ Tetralogy of Fallot consists of four separate defects: ventricular septal defect, overriding aorta, pulmonary stenosis, and right ventricular hypertrophy.   (PED)

■ The goal of crisis intervention is to restore the person to a precrisis level of functioning and order. **(M-S)**

■ According to the *DSM-IV,* bipolar II disorder is characterized by at least one manic episode that's accompanied by hypomania. **(PSY)**

■ Congenital heart defects are classified as cyanotic or acyanotic. **(PED)**

■ Nephrotic syndrome causes proteinuria, hypoalbuminemia, and edema, and sometimes hematuria, hypertension, and a decreased glomerular filtration rate. **(M-S)**

■ Acute glomerulonephritis, the most common noninfectious renal disease of childhood, is commonly caused by a reaction to streptococcal infection. **(PED)**

■ Hydrocephalus may be congenital or may be caused by a tumor, infection, or hemorrhage. **(PED)**

■ *Hyperpyrexia* is extreme elevation in temperature above 106° F (41.1° C). **(FND)**

■ Bowel sounds may be heard over a hernia, but not over a hydrocele. **(M-S)**

■ S_1 is decreased in first-degree heart block. S_2 is decreased in aortic stenosis. **(M-S)**

■ Gas in the colon may cause tympany in the right upper quadrant, obscure liver dullness, and lead to falsely decreased estimates of liver size. **(M-S)**

■ In ataxia caused by loss of position sense, vision compensates for the sensory loss. The patient stands well with the eyes open, but loses balance when they're closed (positive Romberg test result). **(M-S)**

■ Inability to recognize numbers when drawn on the hand with the blunt end of a pen suggests a lesion in the sensory cortex. **(M-S)**

■ Dilated scalp veins indicate long-standing increased intracranial pressure. **(PED)**

■ The nurse can use silence and active listening to promote interactions with a depressed patient. **(PSY)**

- Separation anxiety is a major source of stress for a hospitalized toddler. (PED)

- A major developmental task for a woman during the first trimester of pregnancy is accepting the pregnancy. (MAT)

- A psychiatric patient with a substance abuse problem and a major psychiatric disorder has a dual diagnosis. (PSY)

- During the late stage of multiple myeloma, the patient should be protected against pathological fractures as a result of osteoporosis. (M-S)

- Tricyclic antidepressants such as amitriptyline (Elavil) shouldn't be administered to patients with narrow-angle glaucoma, benign prostatic hypertrophy, or coronary artery disease. (M-S)

- Unlike formula, breast milk offers the benefit of maternal antibodies. (MAT)

- When a patient is readmitted to a mental health unit, the nurse should assess compliance with medication orders. (PSY)

- When the nurse performs chest percussion therapy on a child, percussions (clapping) should be confined to the area around the rib cage. (PED)

- Pulmonary embolism is characterized by a sudden, sharp, stabbing pain in the chest; dyspnea; decreased breath sounds; and crackles or a pleural friction rub on auscultation. (M-S)

- Most poisonings in children younger than age 6 occur when the child takes a substance orally. (PED)

- Obesity is the most common nutritional problem in children. (PED)

- Clinical manifestations of cardiac tamponade are hypotension and jugular vein distention. (M-S)

- To avoid further damage, the nurse shouldn't induce vomiting in a patient who has swallowed a corrosive chemical, such as oven cleaner, drain cleaner, or kerosene. (M-S)

- A brilliant red reflex excludes most serious defects of the cornea, aqueous chamber, lens, and vitreous chamber. (M-S)

- Preschool children commonly stutter because their vocabulary is increasing more quickly than their ability to produce words. This dysfluency in speech pattern is a common characteristic of language development. **(PED)**

- In answering parents' questions about their child's condition, the nurse should use clear, simple explanations. **(PED)**

- Oral hypoglycemic agents stimulate the islets of Langerhans to produce insulin. **(M-S)**

- Alcohol potentiates the effects of tricyclic antidepressants. **(PSY)**

- Spontaneous rupture of the membranes increases the risk of a prolapsed umbilical cord. **(MAT)**

- A clinical manifestation of a prolapsed umbilical cord is variable decelerations. **(MAT)**

- By age 3, a child should be able to stand on one foot. **(PED)**

- *Flight of ideas* is movement from one topic to another without any discernible connection. **(PSY)**

- An 8-month-old infant engages in imitating words. **(PED)**

- Infants with congenital heart defects are at increased risk for heart failure. **(PED)**

- Infants with congenital heart defects should be given small, frequent feedings. The typical schedule is every 3 hours instead of the usual every 4 hours. **(PED)**

- To treat wound dehiscence, the nurse should help the patient to lie in a supine position; cover the protruding intestine with moist, sterile, normal saline packs; and change the packs frequently to keep the area moist. **(M-S)**

- When administering drugs or other forms of treatment to a child, the nurse should allow the child to make choices when appropriate. Making choices allows the child to exercise a certain degree of control and autonomy. **(PED)**

- Milk is high in sodium and low in iron. **(FND)**

While a patient is receiving an I.V. nitroglycerin drip, the nurse should monitor his blood pressure every 15 minutes to detect hypotension.

(M-S)

Conduct disorder is manifested by extreme behavior, such as hurting people and animals. (PSY)

A pacifier shouldn't be given to a neonate who is in the learning stage of breast-feeding. (PED)

Any type of fluid loss can trigger a crisis in a patient with sickle cell anemia. (M-S)

The patient should rinse his mouth after using a corticosteroid inhaler to avoid steroid residue and reduce oral fungal infections. (M-S)

During the "tension-building" phase of an abusive relationship, the abused individual feels helpless. (PSY)

To build trust, the infant needs consistent care, love, and human touch.

(PED)

When caring for a child who is in traction, the nurse should make sure that the body is in alignment, especially the shoulders, hips, and legs.

(PED)

In an infant, signs of impending airway obstruction include increased pulse and respiratory rate; substernal, suprasternal, and intercostal retractions; nasal flaring; and restlessness. (PED)

A patient with low levels of triiodothyronine and thyroxine may have fatigue, lethargy, cold intolerance, constipation, and decreased libido.

(M-S)

During a sickle cell crisis, treatment includes pain management, hydration, and bed rest. (M-S)

When a patient expresses concern about a health-related issue, before addressing the concern, the nurse should assess the patient's level of knowledge. (FND)

The most effective way to reduce a fever is to administer an antipyretic, which lowers the temperature set point. (FND)

■ The preferred treatment of hydrocephalus is the placement of a ventriculoperitoneal shunt to drain the cerebrospinal fluid from the ventricles to an extracranial compartment, usually the peritoneum.   (PED)

■ If parents report that their child holds his breath during tantrums, the nurse should advise the parents that this behavior won't harm the child.   (PED)

■ When a patient is ill, it's essential for the members of his family to maintain communication about his health needs.   (FND)

■ *Ethnocentrism* is the universal belief that one's way of life is superior to others'.   (FND)

■ When a nurse is communicating with a patient through an interpreter, the nurse should speak to the patient and the interpreter.   (FND)

■ In accordance with the "hot-cold" system used by some Mexicans, Puerto Ricans, and other Hispanic and Latino groups, most foods, beverages, herbs, and drugs are described as "cold."   (FND)

■ *Prejudice* is a hostile attitude toward individuals of a particular group.   (FND)

■ *Discrimination* is preferential treatment of individuals of a particular group. It's usually discussed in a negative sense.   (FND)

■ In the emergency treatment of an alcohol-intoxicated patient, determining the blood-alcohol level is paramount in determining the amount of medication that the patient needs.   (PSY)

■ A patient who is hyperventilating should rebreathe into a paper bag to increase the retention of carbon dioxide.   (M-S)

■ Side effects of the antidepressant fluoxetine (Prozac) include diarrhea, decreased libido, weight loss, and dry mouth.   (PSY)

■ Chorea is a major clinical manifestation of central nervous system involvement caused by rheumatic fever.   (M-S)

■ Chorea causes constant jerky, uncontrolled movements; fidgeting; twisting; grimacing; and loss of bowel and bladder control.   (M-S)

- Before electroconvulsive therapy, the patient is given the skeletal muscle relaxant succinylcholine (Anectine) by I.V. administration. **(PSY)**

- Severe diarrhea can cause electrolyte deficiencies and metabolic acidosis. **(M-S)**

- Children with acute glomerulonephritis with edema, oliguria, azotemia, and hypertension usually must restrict their intake of sodium, protein, fluids, and potassium. **(PED)**

- Increased gastric motility interferes with the absorption of oral drugs. **(FND)**

- During labor, to relieve supine hypotension manifested by nausea and vomiting and paleness, turn the patient on her left side. **(MAT)**

- To reduce the risk of hypercalcemia in a patient with metastatic bone cancer, the nurse should help the patient ambulate, promote fluid intake to dilute urine, and limit the patient's oral intake of calcium. **(M-S)**

- An infant who is receiving oxygen through a nasal cannula should be monitored for mouth breathing. **(PED)**

- Negativism is a normal sign of increasing autonomy in a toddler. Parents should react with patience and humor and should avoid head-on confrontations with the child. **(PED)**

- Pain associated with a myocardial infarction usually is described as "pressure" or as a "heavy" or "squeezing" sensation in the midsternal area. The patient may report that the pain feels as though someone is standing on his chest or as though an elephant is sitting on his chest. **(M-S)**

- When a psychotic patient is admitted to an inpatient facility, the primary concern is safety, followed by the establishment of trust. **(PSY)**

- The American Academy of Pediatrics recommends introducing one food at a time to an infant. The first food is cereal, usually rice. **(PED)**

- Calcium and phosphorus levels are elevated until hyperparathyroidism is stabilized. **(M-S)**

- The three phases of the therapeutic relationship are orientation, working, and termination. **(FND)**

Patients often exhibit resistive and challenging behaviors in the orientation phase of the therapeutic relationship.   (FND)

Bronchopulmonary dysplasia is an iatrogenic disease that's caused by intubation and ventilation.   (PED)

After age 4 months, an infant should receive supplemental iron. (PED)

Abdominal assessment is performed in the following order: inspection, auscultation, palpation, and percussion.   (FND)

An effective way to decrease the risk of suicide is to make a suicide contract with the patient for a specified period of time.   (PSY)

The pain associated with carpal tunnel syndrome is caused by entrapment of the median nerve at the wrist.   (M-S)

A depressed patient should be given sufficient portions of his favorite foods, but shouldn't be overwhelmed with too much food.   (PSY)

Pancreatic enzyme replacement enhances the absorption of protein.
                                                                    (M-S)

Laminectomy with spinal fusion is performed to relieve pressure on the spinal nerves and stabilize the spine.   (M-S)

A transection injury of the spinal cord at any level causes paralysis below the level of the lesion.   (M-S)

Toilet sitting can begin at 18 months.   (PED)

To leave room for other nutritious food, toddlers shouldn't drink more than 24 ounces of milk daily.   (PED)

Children age 7 and older can use patient-controlled analgesia.   (PED)

If the ovum is fertilized by a spermatozoon carrying a Y chromosome, a male zygote is formed.   (MAT)

If the ovum is fertilized by a spermatozoon carrying an X chromosome, a female zygote is formed.   (MAT)

Implantation occurs when the cellular walls of the blastocyte implants itself in the endometrium, usually 7 to 9 days after fertilization.   (MAT)

▨ Heart development in the embryo begins at 2 to 4 weeks and is complete by the end of the embryonic stage. **(MAT)**

▨ To determine bone age, X-rays of the tarsals and carpals are obtained to determine the degree of ossification. This technique is used primarily when the child is shorter or taller than expected for his chronological age. **(PED)**

▨ To determine the adjusted, or correct, age of an infant who was born prematurely, the nurse should take the chronological age and subtract the number of weeks that the infant was born prematurely. **(PED)**

▨ When measuring blood pressure in a neonate, the nurse should select a cuff that's no less than one-half and no more than two-thirds the length of the extremity that's used. **(FND)**

▨ An infant should be weaned from the bottle between the ages of 10 and 12 months. **(PED)**

▨ When administering an oral drug to an infant, the nurse should instill the drug along the side of the tongue to prevent gagging and expulsion of the drug. **(PED)**

▨ When administering a drug by Z-track, the nurse shouldn't use the same needle that was used to draw the drug into the syringe because doing so could stain the skin. **(FND)**

▨ Sites for intradermal injection include the inner arm, the upper chest, and on the back, under the scapula. **(FND)**

▨ For pulseless ventricular tachycardia, the patient should be defibrillated immediately, with 200 joules, 300 joules, and then 360 joules given in rapid succession. **(M-S)**

▨ Pleural friction rub is heard in pleurisy, pneumonia, and plural infarction. **(M-S)**

▨ Wheezes are heard in emphysema, foreign body obstruction, and asthma. **(M-S)**

▨ Rhonchi are heard in pneumonia, emphysema, bronchitis, and bronchiectasis. **(M-S)**

■ Crackles are heard in pulmonary edema, pneumonia, and pulmonary fibrosis. (M-S)

■ Clinical manifestations of epiglottitis are constant drooling, agitation or restlessness, and the absence of spontaneous cough. (PED)

■ The nurse shouldn't take an oral temperature or examine the throat of child who is suspected of having epiglottitis. (PED)

■ Clinical manifestations of croup are hoarseness, a barking or brassy cough, respiratory distress, and stridor. (PED)

■ The electrocardiogram of a patient with heart failure shows ventricular hypertrophy. (M-S)

■ A decrease in the potassium level decreases the effectiveness of cardiac glycosides, increases the possibility of digoxin toxicity, and can cause fatal cardiac arrhythmias. (M-S)

■ A crying infant must be calmed before his vital signs are obtained. (PED)

■ A 12-lead electrocardiogram reading should be obtained during a myocardial infarction or an anginal attack. (M-S)

■ The primary difference between angina and the symptoms of a myocardial infarction (MI) is that angina can be relieved by rest or nitroglycerin administration. The symptoms of an MI aren't relieved with rest, and the pain can last 30 minutes or longer. (M-S)

■ Calcium channel blockers include verapamil (Calan), diltiazem hydrochloride (Cardizem), nifedipine (Procardia), and nicardipine hydrochloride (Cardene). (M-S)

■ After a myocardial infarction, electrocardiograph changes include elevations of the Q wave and ST segment. (M-S)

■ Antiarrhythmic agents include quinidine gluconate (Quinaglute), lidocaine hydrochloride, and procainamide hydrochloride (Pronestyl). (M-S)

■ Angiotensin-converting enzyme inhibitors include captopril and enalapril maleate (Vasotec). (M-S)

▒ After a myocardial infarction, the patient should avoid stressful activities and situations, such as exertion, hot or cold temperatures, and emotional stress. **(M-S)**

▒ Antihypertensive drugs include hydralazine hydrochloride (Apresoline) and methyldopa (Aldomet). **(M-S)**

▒ When evaluating whether an answer on an examination is correct, the nurse should consider whether the action that's described promotes autonomy (independence), safety, self-esteem, and a sense of belonging. **(FND)**

▒ According to Piaget, between the ages of 2 and 7, the child is in the ego-centric stage and isn't particularly concerned about rules. **(PED)**

▒ When answering a question on the NCLEX examination, the student should consider the cue (the stimulus for a thought) and the inference (the thought) to determine whether the inference is correct. When in doubt, the nurse should select an answer that indicates the need for further information to eliminate ambiguity. For example, the patient complains of chest pain (the stimulus for the thought) and the nurse infers that the patient is having cardiac pain (the thought). In this case, the nurse hasn't confirmed whether the pain is cardiac. It would be more appropriate to make further assessments. **(FND)**

▒ *Veracity* is truth and is an essential component of a therapeutic relationship between a health care provider and his patient. **(FND)**

▒ *Beneficence* is the duty to do no harm and the duty to do good. There's an obligation in patient care to do no harm and an equal obligation to assist the patient. **(FND)**

▒ *Nonmaleficence* is the duty to do no harm. **(FND)**

▒ Frye's ABCDE cascade provides a framework for prioritizing care by identifying the most important treatment concerns. **(FND)**

▒ A = Airway. This category includes everything that affects a patent airway, including a foreign object, fluid from an upper respiratory infection, and edema from trauma or an allergic reaction. **(FND)**

B = Breathing. This category includes everything that affects the breathing pattern, including hyperventilation or hypoventilation and abnormal breathing patterns, such as Korsakoff's, Biot's, or Cheyne-Stokes respiration. **(FND)**

C = Circulation. This category includes everything that affects the circulation, including fluid and electrolyte disturbances and disease processes that affect cardiac output. **(FND)**

D = Disease processes. If the patient has no problem with the airway, breathing, or circulation, then the nurse should evaluate the disease processes, giving priority to the disease process that poses the greatest immediate risk. For example, if a patient has terminal cancer and hypoglycemia, hypoglycemia is a more immediate concern. **(FND)**

E = Everything else. This category includes such issues as writing an incident report and completing the patient chart. When evaluating needs, this category is never the highest priority. **(FND)**

When answering a question on an NCLEX examination, the basic rule is "assess before action." The student should evaluate each possible answer carefully. Usually, several answers reflect the implementation phase of nursing and one or two reflect the assessment phase. In this case, the best choice is an assessment response unless a specific course of action is clearly indicated. **(FND)**

Masturbation is most common at age 4 and during adolescence. **(PED)**

Modeling is a form of behavior in which children imitate the behavior of a significant other, such as a parent. **(PED)**

Rule utilitarianism is known as the "greatest good for the greatest number of people" theory. **(FND)**

Egalitarian theory emphasizes that equal access to goods and services must be provided to the less fortunate by an affluent society. **(FND)**

Active euthanasia is actively helping a person to die. **(FND)**

Brain death is irreversible cessation of all brain function. **(FND)**

Passive euthanasia is stopping the therapy that's sustaining life. **(FND)**

- Both parents must have a recessive gene for the offspring to inherit the gene. **(M-S)**

- A third-party payer is an insurance company. **(FND)**

- Utilization review is performed to determine whether the care provided to a patient was appropriate and cost-effective. **(FND)**

- A *value cohort* is a group of people who experienced an out-of-the-ordinary event that shaped their values. **(FND)**

- *Voluntary euthanasia* is actively helping a patient to die at the patient's request. **(FND)**

- A dominant gene is a gene that only needs to be present in one parent to have a 50–50 chance of affecting each offspring. **(M-S)**

- Bananas, citrus fruits, and potatoes are good sources of potassium. **(FND)**

- Good sources of magnesium include fish, nuts, and grains. **(FND)**

- Bronchodilators dilate the bronchioles and relax bronchiolar smooth muscle. **(M-S)**

- The primary function of aldosterone is sodium reabsorption. **(M-S)**

- The goal of positive end-expiratory pressure is to achieve adequate arterial oxygenation without using a toxic level of inspired oxygen or compromising cardiac output. **(M-S)**

- Prolonged use of oxygen in the neonate may cause retrolental fibroplasia and may cause blindness. Arterial oxygen saturation usually is maintained at less than 94%. **(PED)**

- Beef, oysters, shrimp, scallops, spinach, beets, and greens are good sources of iron. **(FND)**

- Furosemide (Lasix) is a loop diuretic. Its onset of action is 30 to 60 minutes, peak is achieved at 1 to 2 hours, and duration is 6 to 8 hours for the I.M. or oral route. **(M-S)**

- Pregnancy, myocardial infarction, GI bleeding, bleeding disorders, and hemorrhoids are contraindications to manual removal of fecal impaction. **(M-S)**

■ Ambulation is the best method to prevent postoperative atelectasis. Other measures include incentive spirometry and turning, coughing, and breathing deeply. (M-S)

■ *Intrathecal injection* is administering a drug through the spine. (FND)

■ The blood urea nitrogen test and the creatinine clearance test measure how effectively the kidneys excrete these respective substances. (M-S)

■ The nurse should assess the depressed patient for suicidal ideation. (PSY)

■ The first sign of respiratory distress or compromise is restlessness. (M-S)

■ When a patient asks a question or makes a statement that's emotionally charged, the nurse should respond to the emotion behind the statement or question rather than to what's being said or asked. (FND)

■ The antidote for magnesium sulfate overdose is calcium gluconate 10%. (M-S)

■ The antidote for heparin overdose is protamine sulfate. (M-S)

■ Methergine stimulates uterine contractions. (MAT)

■ An allergic reaction to a blood transfusion may include flushing, urticaria, wheezing, and a rash. If the patient has any of these signs of a reaction, the nurse should stop the transfusion immediately, keep the vein open with normal saline, and notify the physician. (M-S)

■ Discharge instructions to the parents of a child with asthma include instructing the child and parent to use a peak flow monitor to track the peak expiratory flow readings. (PED)

■ When assessing a child with Wilms' tumor, the nurse should avoid palpating the abdomen and thus the mass. (PED)

■ A patient taking digoxin and furosemide (Lasix) should call the physician if he experiences muscle weakness. (M-S)

■ A patient with basal cell carcinoma should avoid exposure to the sun during the hottest time of day (between 10 a.m. and 3 p.m.). (M-S)

■ A clinical manifestation of acute pain is diaphoresis. (M-S)

- The steps of the trajectory-nursing model are as follows:
  - Step 1: Identifying the trajectory phase
  - Step 2: Identifying the problems and establishing goals
  - Step 3: Establishing a plan to meet the goals
  - Step 4: Identifying factors that facilitate or hinder attainment of the goals
  - Step 5: Implementing interventions
  - Step 6: Evaluating the effectiveness of the interventions   (FND)

- A Hindu patient is likely to request a vegetarian diet.   (FND)

- *Gardnerella* vaginitis is a type of bacterial vaginosis that causes a thin, watery, milklike discharge that has a fishy odor.   (M-S)

- If a child has a blood lead level greater than 45 mg/dl, the physician may order chelation therapy (EDTA).   (PED)

- The administration of folic acid during the early stages of gestation may prevent neural tube defects.   (MAT)

- A patient who is taking Flagyl (metronidazole) shouldn't consume alcoholic beverages or use preparations that contain alcohol because they may cause a disulfiram-like reaction (flushing, headache, vomiting, and abdominal pain).   (M-S)

- With advanced maternal age, a common genetic problem is Down syndrome.   (MAT)

- With early maternal age, cephalopelvic disproportion commonly occurs.   (MAT)

- During the administration of transcutaneous electrical nerve stimulation, the patient feels a tingling sensation.   (M-S)

- In the early postpartum period, the fundus should be midline at the umbilicus.   (MAT)

- *Pain threshold*, or pain sensation, is the initial point at which a patient feels pain.   (FND)

- In patients with glaucoma, the head of the bed should be elevated in the semi-Fowler position or as ordered after surgery to promote drainage of aqueous humor.   (M-S)

Postoperative care after peripheral iridectomy includes administering drugs (steroids and cycloplegics) as prescribed to decrease inflammation and dilate the pupils. **(M-S)**

The difference between acute pain and chronic pain is its duration. **(FND)**

Referred pain is pain that's felt at a site other than its origin. **(FND)**

The youngest age at which it's appropriate to use the face scale to indicate the severity of pain is age 3. **(PED)**

Alleviating pain by performing a back massage is consistent with the gate control theory. **(FND)**

Retinopathy refers to changes in retinal capillaries that decrease blood flow to the retina and lead to ischemia, hemorrhage, and retinal detachment. **(M-S)**

Kegel exercises are recommended after surgery to improve the tone of the sphincter and pelvic muscles. **(M-S)**

Romberg's test is a test for balance or gait. **(FND)**

One of the treatments for trichomoniasis vaginalis is metronidazole (Flagyl), which must be prescribed for the patient and the patient's sexual partner. **(M-S)**

Pain seems more intense at night because the patient isn't distracted by daily activities. **(FND)**

A rubella vaccine shouldn't be given to a pregnant woman. The vaccine can be administered after delivery, but the patient should be instructed to avoid becoming pregnant for 3 months. **(MAT)**

A 16-year-old girl who is pregnant is at risk for having a low-birth-weight neonate. **(MAT)**

A common symptom after cataract laser surgery is blurred vision. **(M-S)**

A patient with acute open-angle glaucoma may see halos around lights. **(M-S)**

An Asian patient with diabetes mellitus usually can drink ginseng tea. **(M-S)**

- Older patients commonly don't report pain because of fear of treatment, lifestyle changes, or dependency. **(FND)**

- To prevent otitis externa, the patient should keep the ears dry when bathing. **(M-S)**

- Patients who receive prolonged high doses of I.V. furosemide (Lasix) should be assessed for tinnitus and hearing loss. **(M-S)**

- The mother's Rh factor should be determined before an amniocentesis is performed. **(MAT)**

- Maternal hypotension is a complication of spinal block. **(MAT)**

- The treatment for toxic shock syndrome is I.V. fluid administration to restore blood volume and pressure and antibiotic therapy to eliminate infection. **(M-S)**

- In patients with glaucoma, beta-adrenergic blockers facilitate the outflow of aqueous humor. **(M-S)**

- No pork or pork products are allowed in a Muslim diet. **(FND)**

- Two goals of *Healthy People 2010* are:
  1. Help individuals of all ages to increase the quality of life and the number of years of optimal health
  2. Eliminate health disparities among different segments of the population. **(FND)**

- A community nurse is serving as a patient's advocate if she tells a malnourished patient to go to a meal program at a local park. **(FND)**

- After delivery, if the fundus is boggy and deviated to the right side, the patient should empty her bladder. **(MAT)**

- A man who loses one testicle should still be able to father a child. **(M-S)**

- If a patient isn't following his treatment plan, the nurse should first ask why. **(FND)**

- Falls are the leading cause of injury in elderly people. **(FND)**

- Native Americans are particularly susceptible to diabetes mellitus.**(M-S)**

- Blacks are particularly susceptible to hypertension. **(M-S)**

Women with the greatest risk for cervical cancer are those whose mothers had cervical cancer, followed by those whose female siblings had cervical cancer.   (M-S)

A postmenopausal woman should perform breast self-examination on the same day each month, for example, on the same day of the month as her birthday.   (M-S)

Middle-ear hearing loss usually results from otosclerosis.   (M-S)

After testicular surgery, the patient should use an ice pack for comfort.   (M-S)

Primary prevention is true prevention. Examples are immunizations, weight control, and smoking cessation.   (FND)

Secondary prevention is early detection. Examples include purified protein derivative (PPD), breast self-examination, testicular self-examination, and chest X-ray.   (FND)

Tertiary prevention is treatment to prevent long-term complications.
                                                                              (FND)

Before providing a specimen for a sperm count, the patient should avoid ejaculation for 48 to 72 hours.   (MAT)

A patient indicates that he's coming to terms with having a chronic disease when he says, "I'm never going to get any better."   (FND)

A patient with chronic open-angle glaucoma has tunnel vision. The nurse must be careful to place items directly in front of him so that he can see them.   (M-S)

On noticing religious artifacts and literature on a patient's night stand, a culturally aware nurse would ask the patient the meaning of the items.
                                                                              (FND)

A Mexican patient may request the intervention of a curandero, or faith healer, who involves the family in healing the patient.   (FND)

The hormone human chorionic gonadotropin is a marker for pregnancy.
                                                                              (MAT)

Painless vaginal bleeding during the last trimester of pregnancy may indicate placenta previa.   (MAT)

- Clinical signs of bacterial pneumonia include shaking, chills, fever, and a cough that produces purulent sputum.   **(M-S)**

- During the transition phase of labor, the woman usually is irritable and restless.   **(MAT)**

- Clinical manifestations of flail chest include paradoxical movement of the involved chest wall, dyspnea, pain, and cyanosis.   **(M-S)**

- Right-sided cardiac function is assessed by evaluating central venous pressure.   **(M-S)**

- A patient with a pacemaker should immediately report an increase in the pulse rate or a slowing of the pulse rate of more than 4 to 5 beats/minute.   **(M-S)**

- Dizziness, fainting, palpitation, hiccups, and chest pain indicate pacemaker failure.   **(M-S)**

- Leukemia causes easy fatigability, generalized malaise, and pallor. **(M-S)**

- After cardiac catheterization, the puncture, or cutdown, site should be monitored for hematoma formation.   **(M-S)**

- Because women with diabetes have a higher incidence of birth anomalies than women without diabetes, an alpha-fetoprotein level may be ordered at 15 to 17 weeks' gestation.   **(MAT)**

- Kussmaul's breathing is associated with diabetic ketoacidosis.   **(M-S)**

- If the nurse notices water in a ventilator tube, she should remove the water from the tube and reconnect it.   **(M-S)**

- Tamoxifen is an antineoplastic drug that's used to treat breast cancer.   **(M-S)**

- The adverse effects of vincristine (Oncovin) include alopecia, nausea, and vomiting.   **(M-S)**

- To avoid puncturing the placenta, a vaginal examination shouldn't be performed on a pregnant patient who is bleeding.   **(MAT)**

- A patient who has postpartum hemorrhage caused by uterine atony should be given oxytocin as prescribed.   **(MAT)**

- Emphysema is characterized by destruction of the alveoli, enlargement of the distal air spaces, and breakdown of the alveolar walls. (M-S)

- To keep secretions thin, the patient who has emphysema should increase his fluid intake to approximately 2.5 L/day. (M-S)

- The clinical manifestations of asthma are wheezing, dyspnea, hypoxemia, diaphoresis, and increased heart and respiratory rate. (M-S)

- *Extrinsic asthma* is an antigen–antibody reaction to allergens, such as pollen, animal, dander, feathers, foods, house dust, or mites. (M-S)

- Laceration of the vagina, cervix, or perineum produces bright red bleeding that often comes in spurts. The bleeding is continuous, even when the fundus is firm. (MAT)

- To stimulate the rooting reflex and promote feeding of a bottle-fed infant, the nurse should stroke his cheek. (PED)

- After endoscopy is performed, the nurse should assess the patient for hemoptysis. (M-S)

- Increased urine output is an indication that a hypertensive crisis has resolved. (M-S)

- After radical mastectomy, the patient should be positioned with the affected arm on pillows with the hand elevated and aligned with the arm. (M-S)

- After pneumonectomy, the patient should perform arm exercises to prevent frozen shoulder. (M-S)

- Right-sided heart failure causes edema, distended neck veins, nocturia, and weakness. (M-S)

- Left-sided heart failure causes crackles, coughing, tachycardia, and fatigability. (Think of *L* to remember Left and Lungs.) (M-S)

- Cardiac glycosides increase contractility and cardiac output. (M-S)

- Adverse effects of cardiac glycosides include cardiac disturbance, headache, hypotension, GI symptoms, blurred vision, and yellow-green halos around lights. (M-S)

▪ A patient who is receiving anticoagulant therapy should take acetaminophen (Tylenol) instead of aspirin for pain relief.   (M-S)

▪ Adequate humidification is important after laryngectomy. At home, the
patient can use pans of water or a cool mist vaporizer, especially in the
bedroom.   (M-S)

▪ Late symptoms of renal cancer include hematuria, flank pain, and a palpable mass in the flank.   (M-S)

▪ Heparin is given subcutaneously, usually in the lower abdominal fat pad.
    (M-S)

▪ In a patient with sickle cell anemia, warm packs should be used over the
extremities to relieve pain. Cold packs may stimulate vasoconstriction
and cause further ischemia. The extremities should be placed on pillows
for comfort.   (M-S)

▪ Sickle cell crisis causes sepsis (fever greater than 102° F [38.9° C],
meningeal irritation, tachypnea, tachycardia, and hypotension) and vaso-
occlusive crisis (severe pain) with hypoxia (partial pressure of arterial
oxygen of less than 70 mm Hg).   (M-S)

▪ In an infant, the normal hemoglobin value is 12 g/dl.   (FND)

▪ Adverse effects of digoxin include headache, weakness, vision disturbances, anorexia, and GI upset.   (M-S)

▪ To perform a tuberculosis test, a 26-gauge needle is used with a 1-ml syringe.   (M-S)

▪ The nitrogen balance estimates the difference between the intake and use
of protein.   (FND)

▪ Respiratory failure occurs when mucus blocks the alveoli or the airways
of the lungs.   (M-S)

▪ The patient should be instructed not to cough during thoracentesis.
    (M-S)

▪ Hot compresses can help to relieve breast tenderness after breast-feeding.
    (MAT)

A patient who has thrombophlebitis should be placed in the Trendelenburg position. (M-S)

Symptoms of *Pneumocystis carinii* pneumonia include dyspnea and nonproductive cough. (M-S)

To counteract vitamin B_1 deficiency, a patient who has pernicious anemia should eat meat and animal products. (M-S)

A patient who is on a ventilator and becomes restless should undergo suctioning. (M-S)

A premature neonate has a decrease in surfactant that leads to decreased oxygen consumption. (PED)

Autologous bone marrow transplantation doesn't cause graft-versus-host disease. (M-S)

A patient who has mild thrombophlebitis is likely to have mild cramping on exertion. (M-S)

If the first attempt to perform colostomy irrigation is unsuccessful, the procedure is repeated with normal saline solution. (M-S)

The fundus of a postpartum patient is massaged to stimulate contraction of the uterus and prevent hemorrhage. (MAT)

Breast enlargement, or gynecomastia, is an adverse effect of estrogen therapy. (M-S)

In a patient who has leukemia, a low platelet count may lead to hemorrhage. (M-S)

After radical neck dissection, the immediate concern is respiratory distress as a result of tracheal edema. (M-S)

Naloxone (Narcan) is given to a neonate who is experiencing the effects of maternal narcotic administration during labor and delivery. (PED)

In a neonate who is large for gestational age, the serum glucose level should be measured. (PED)

A mother who has a positive human immunodeficiency virus test result shouldn't breast-feed her infant. (MAT)

▓ After radical mastectomy, the patient's arm should be elevated to prevent lymphedema. (M-S)

▓ Hypoventilation causes respiratory acidosis. (M-S)

▓ The high Fowler position is the best position for a patient who has orthopnea. (M-S)

▓ To obtain a urine specimen in an infant, a specimen bag (Hollister U bag) is used. (PED)

▓ A transient ischemic attack affects sensory and motor function and may cause diplopia, dysphagia, aphasia, and ataxia. (M-S)

▓ After mastectomy, the patient should squeeze a ball with the hand on the affected side. (M-S)

▓ Cholestyramine (Questran), which is used to reduce the serum cholesterol level, may cause constipation. (M-S)

▓ Dinoprostone (Cervidil) is used to ripen the cervix. (MAT)

▓ Glucocorticoid, or steroid, therapy may mask the signs of infection. (M-S)

▓ After the death of a child, the parents should be allowed to stay with the deceased for as long as they wish. (PED)

▓ Breast-feeding of a premature neonate born at 32 weeks' gestation can be accomplished if the mother expresses milk and feeds the neonate by gavage. (MAT)

▓ Melanoma is most commonly seen in light-skinned people who work or spend time outdoors. (M-S)

▓ A patient who has a pacemaker should take his pulse at the same time every day. (M-S)

▓ A patient who has stomatitis should rinse his mouth with mouthwash frequently. (M-S)

▓ An adverse effect of theophylline administration is tachycardia. (M-S)

▓ The treatment for laryngotracheobronchitis includes postural drainage before meals. (M-S)

After radical neck dissection, a high priority is providing a means of communication. (M-S)

A high-fat diet that includes red meat is a contributing factor for colorectal cancer. (M-S)

After a modified radical mastectomy, the patient should be placed in the semi-Fowler position, with the arm placed on a pillow. (M-S)

A young child is sedated before cardiac catheterization is performed. (PED)

Knifelike, stabbing pain in the chest may indicate pulmonary embolism. (M-S)

Esophageal cancer is associated with excessive alcohol consumption. (M-S)

If a pregnant patient's rubella titer is less than 1:8, she should be immunized after delivery. (MAT)

The administration of oxytocin (Pitocin) is stopped if the contractions are 90 seconds or longer. (MAT)

For an extramural delivery (one that takes place outside of a normal delivery center), the priorities for care of the neonate include maintaining a patent airway, supporting efforts to breathe, monitoring vital signs, and maintaining adequate body temperature. (MAT)

When a neonate receives phototherapy with a fiberoptic light, it isn't necessary to cover his eyes or genitals. (PED)

A patient who has pancytopenia and is undergoing chemotherapy may experience hemorrhage and infection. (M-S)

A grade I tumor is encapsulated and grows by expansion. (M-S)

Subinvolution may occur if the bladder is distended after delivery. (MAT)

The nurse must place identification bands on both the mother and the neonate before they leave the delivery room. (MAT)

Cancer of the pancreas causes anorexia, weight loss, and jaundice. (M-S)

■ Erythromycin is given at birth to prevent ophthalmia neonatorum.

(MAT)

■ Most of the absorption of water occurs in the large intestine.   (FND)

■ Most nutrients are absorbed in the small intestine.   (FND)

■ Prolonged gastric suctioning can cause metabolic alkalosis.   (M-S)

■ To measure the amount of residual urine, the nurse performs straight catheterization after the patient voids.   (M-S)

■ Dexamethasone (Decadron) is a steroidal anti-inflammatory agent that's used to treat brain tumors.   (M-S)

■ Long-term reduction in the delivery of oxygen to the kidneys causes an increase in erythropoiesis.   (M-S)

■ When assessing a patient's eating habits, the nurse should ask, "What have you eaten in the last 24 hours?"   (FND)

■ A vegan diet should include an abundant supply of fiber.   (FND)

■ To facilitate emptying of the stomach after feeding, the neonate is positioned on his right side.   (PED)

■ A patient who subsists on canned foods and canned fish is at risk for sodium imbalance (*hypernatremia*).   (M-S)

■ Clinical signs and symptoms of hypoxia include confusion, diaphoresis, changes in blood pressure, tachycardia, and tachypnea.   (M-S)

■ Red meat can cause a false-positive result on fecal occult blood test.

(M-S)

■ Carbon monoxide replaces hemoglobin in the red blood cells, decreasing the amount of oxygen in the tissue.   (M-S)

■ Alkaline urine can result in urinary tract infection.   (M-S)

■ A hypotonic enema softens the feces, distends the colon, and stimulates peristalsis.   (FND)

■ Bladder retraining is effective if it lengthens the intervals between urination.   (M-S)

Cheilosis is caused by riboflavin deficiency. (M-S)

First-morning urine provides the best sample to measure glucose, ketone, pH, and specific gravity values. (FND)

The concentration of oxygen in inspired air is reduced at high altitudes. As a result, dyspnea may occur on exertion. (M-S)

A patient who is receiving enteric feeding should be assessed for abdominal distention. (M-S)

Thiamine deficiency causes neuropathy. (M-S)

A patient who has abdominal distention as a result of flatus can be treated with a carminative enema (Harris flush). (M-S)

Pernicious anemia is caused by a deficiency of vitamin B_{12}, or cobalamin. (M-S)

After a barium enema, the patient is given a laxative. (M-S)

The appropriate I.V. fluid to correct a hypovolemic, or fluid volume, deficit is normal saline solution. (M-S)

Serum albumin deficiency commonly occurs after burn injury. (M-S)

Before giving a gastrostomy feeding, the nurse should inspect the patient's stoma. (M-S)

The most common intestinal bacteria identified in urinary tract infection is *Escherichia coli*. (M-S)

Hyponatremia may occur in a patient who has a high fever and drinks only water. (M-S)

Folic acid deficiency causes muscle weakness as a result of hypoxemia. (M-S)

Dehydration causes increased respiration and heart rate, followed by irritability and fussiness. (M-S)

To induce sleep, the first step is to minimize environmental stimuli. (FND)

■ Before moving a patient, the nurse should assess the patient's physical abilities and ability to understand instructions as well as the amount of strength required to move the patient.   (FND)

■ The nurse should maintain a child's bedtime ritual, such as reading a story or holding a favorite blanket or toy to promote sleep.   (PED)

■ Glucocorticoids can cause an electrolyte imbalance.   (M-S)

■ A decrease in potassium level decreases the effectiveness of cardiac glycosides, increases possible digoxin toxicity, and can cause fatal cardiac arrhythmias.   (M-S)

■ Diuresis can cause decreased absorption of vitamins A, D, E, and K.
(M-S)

■ Protein depletion causes a decrease in lymphocyte count.   (M-S)

■ To lose 1 lb (0.5 kg) in 1 week, the patient must decrease his weekly intake by 3,500 calories (approximately 500 calories daily). To lose 2 lb (1 kg) in 1 week, the patient must decrease his weekly caloric intake by 7,000 calories (approximately 1,000 calories daily).   (FND)

■ To prevent paraphimosis after the insertion of a Foley catheter, the nurse should replace the prepuce.   (M-S)

■ To avoid shearing force injury, a patient who is completely immobile is lifted on a sheet.   (FND)

■ Loop diuretics, such as furosemide (Lasix), decrease plasma levels of potassium and sodium.   (M-S)

■ After pyelography, the patient should drink plenty of fluids to promote the excretion of dye.   (M-S)

■ Potassium should be taken with food and fluids.   (M-S)

■ To insert a catheter from the nose through the trachea for suction, the nurse should ask the patient to swallow.   (FND)

■ Proper measurement of a nasogastric tube is from the corner of the mouth to the ear lobe to the tip of the sternum.   (M-S)

■ Vitamin C is needed for collagen production.   (FND)

Only the patient can describe his pain accurately.   (FND)

Full agonist analgesics include morphine, codeine, meperidine (Demerol), propoxyphene (Darvon), and hydromorphone (Dilaudid).   (M-S)

Buprenorphine (Buprenex) is a partial agonist analgesic.   (M-S)

Cutaneous stimulation creates the release of endorphins that block the transmission of pain stimuli.   (FND)

Patient-controlled anesthesia is a safe method to relieve acute pain caused by surgical incision, traumatic injury, labor and delivery, or cancer.

(FND)

An Asian American or European American typically places distance between himself and others when communicating.   (FND)

The patient who believes in a scientific, or biomedical, approach to health is likely to expect a drug, treatment, or surgery to cure illness.   (FND)

Chronic illnesses occur in very young as well as middle-aged and very old people.   (FND)

The trajectory framework for chronic illness states that preferences about daily life activities affect treatment decisions.   (FND)

Exacerbations of chronic disease usually cause the patient to seek treatment and may lead to hospitalization.   (FND)

School health programs provide cost-effective health care for low-income families and those who have no health insurance.   (FND)

Delusional thought patterns commonly occur during the manic phase of bipolar disorder.   (PSY)

Apathy is typically observed in patients who have schizophrenia. (PSY)

Manipulative behavior is characteristic of a patient who has passive–aggressive personality disorder.   (PSY)

When a patient who has schizophrenia begins to hallucinate, the nurse should redirect the patient to activities that are focused on the here and now.   (PSY)

■ When a patient who is receiving an antipsychotic drug exhibits muscle rigidity and tremors, the nurse should administer an antiparkinsonian drug (for example, Cogentin or Artane) as ordered.   **(PSY)**

■ Poor skin turgor is a clinical manifestation of diabetes insipidus. **(M-S)**

■ A patient who has Addison's disease and is receiving corticosteroid therapy may be at risk for infection.   **(M-S)**

■ To assess a patient for hemorrhage after a thyroidectomy, the nurse should roll the patient onto his side to examine the sides and back of the neck.   **(M-S)**

■ A patient who is receiving hormone therapy for hypothyroidism should take the drug at the same time each day.   **(M-S)**

■ Hyperproteinemia may contribute to the development of hepatic encephalopathy.   **(M-S)**

■ To minimize bleeding in a patient who has liver dysfunction, small-gauge needles are used for injections.   **(M-S)**

■ A patient who has cirrhosis of the liver and ascites should follow a low-sodium diet.   **(M-S)**

■ Before an excretory urography, the nurse must ask the patient whether he's allergic to iodine or shellfish.   **(M-S)**

■ A *buffalo hump* is an abnormal distribution of adipose tissue that occurs in Cushing's syndrome.   **(M-S)**

■ Levothyroxine (Synthroid) is used as replacement therapy in hypothyroidism.   **(M-S)**

■ Acne vulgaris is one result of the hormonal changes of adolescence and is caused by androgenic stimulation of sebum production.   **(PED)**

■ Levothyroxine (Synthroid) treats, but doesn't cure, hypothyroidism and must be taken for the patient's lifetime. It shouldn't be taken with food because food may interfere with its absorption.   **(M-S)**

■ Imipramine (Tofranil) with concomitant use of barbiturates may result in enhanced CNS depression.   **(M-S)**

■ A patient who is receiving levothyroxine (Synthroid) therapy should report tachycardia to the physician.   (M-S)

■ The signs and symptoms of hyperkalemia include muscle weakness, hypotension, shallow respiration, apathy, and anorexia.   (M-S)

■ In a patient with well-controlled diabetes, the 2-hour postprandial blood sugar level may be 139 mg/dl.   (M-S)

■ A patient who has diabetes mellitus should wash his feet daily in warm water and dry them carefully, especially between the toes.   (M-S)

■ Acute pancreatitis causes constant epigastric abdominal pain that radiates to the back and flank and is more intense in the supine position. (M-S)

■ A patient who is receiving lithium (Eskalith) therapy should report diarrhea, vomiting, drowsiness, muscular weakness, or lack of coordination to the physician immediately.   (PSY)

■ The therapeutic serum level of lithium (Eskalith) for maintenance is 0.6 to 1.2 mEq/L.   (PSY)

■ Obsessive-compulsive disorder is an anxiety-related disorder.   (PSY)

■ Al-Anon is a self-help group for families of alcoholics.   (PSY)

■ *Desensitization* is a treatment for phobia, or irrational fear. (PSY)

■ After electroconvulsive therapy, the patient is placed in the lateral position, with the head turned to one side.   (PSY)

■ A *delusion* is a fixed false belief.   (PSY)

■ Giving away personal possessions is a sign of suicidal ideation. Other signs include writing a suicide note or talking about suicide.   (PSY)

■ *Agoraphobia* is fear of open spaces.   (PSY)

■ A person who has paranoid personality disorder projects hostilities onto others.   (PSY)

■ Diabetic neuropathy is a long-term complication of diabetes mellitus.   (M-S)

■ To assess a patient's judgment, the nurse should ask the patient what he would do if he found a stamped, addressed envelope. An appropriate response is that he would mail the envelope.   (PSY)

- After electroconvulsive therapy, the patient should be monitored for post-shock amnesia.   (PSY)

- A mother who continues to perform cardiopulmonary resuscitation after a physician pronounces a child dead is showing denial.   (PSY)

- *Transvestism* is a desire to wear clothes usually worn by members of the opposite sex.   (PSY)

- Portal vein hypertension is associated with liver cirrhosis.   (M-S)

- After thyroidectomy, the nurse should assess the patient for laryngeal damage manifested by hoarseness.   (M-S)

- The patient with hypoparathyroidism has hypocalcemia.   (M-S)

- Tardive dyskinesia causes excessive blinking and unusual movement of the tongue, and involuntary sucking and chewing.   (PSY)

- Trihexyphenidyl (Artane) and benztropine (Cogentin) are administered to counteract extrapyramidal adverse effects.   (PSY)

- To prevent hypertensive crisis, a patient who is taking a monoamine oxidase inhibitor should avoid consuming aged cheese, caffeine, beer, yeast, chocolate, liver, processed foods, and monosodium glutamate.   (PSY)

- Extrapyramidal symptoms include parkinsonism, dystonia, akathisia ("ants in the pants"), and tardive dyskinesia.   (PSY)

- A patient who has chronic pancreatitis should consume a bland, low-fat diet.   (M-S)

- A patient with hepatitis A should be on enteric precautions to prevent the spread of hepatitis A.   (M-S)

- The patient who has liver disease is likely to have jaundice, which is caused by an increased bilirubin level.   (M-S)

- An adverse effect of phenytoin (Dilantin) administration is hyperplasia of the gingiva.   (M-S)

- Protein intake must be monitored in the child who has phenylketonuria.   (PED)

- Hematemesis is a clinical sign of esophageal varices.   (M-S)

Fat destruction is the chemical process that causes ketones to appear in urine.   (M-S)

One theory that supports the use of electroconvulsive therapy suggests that it "resets" the brain circuits to allow normal function.   (PSY)

The glucose tolerance test is the definitive diagnostic test for diabetes.   (M-S)

A patient who has obsessive-compulsive disorder usually recognizes the senselessness of his behavior but is powerless to stop it (ego-dystonia).   (PSY)

Atelectasis and dehiscence are postoperative conditions associated with removal of the gallbladder.   (M-S)

After liver biopsy, the patient should be positioned on his right side, with a pillow placed underneath the liver border.   (M-S)

In helping a patient who has been abused, physical safety is the nurse's first priority.   (PSY)

Pemoline (Cylert) is used to treat attention deficit hyperactivity disorder (ADHD).   (PSY)

Lugol's solution is used to devascularize the gland before thyroidectomy.   (M-S)

Clozapine (Clozaril) is contraindicated in pregnant women and in patients who have severe granulocytopenia or severe central nervous system depression.   (PSY)

Cholecystitis causes low-grade fever, nausea and vomiting, guarding of the right upper quadrant, and biliary pain that radiates to the right scapula.   (M-S)

Early symptoms of liver cirrhosis include fatigue, anorexia, edema of the ankles in the evening, epistaxis, and bleeding gums.   (M-S)

Repression, an unconscious process, is the inability to recall painful or unpleasant thoughts or feelings.   (PSY)

Projection is shifting of unwanted characteristics or shortcomings to others (scapegoat).   (PSY)

The clinical manifestations of diabetes insipidus include polydipsia, polyuria, specific gravity of 1.001 to 1.005, and high serum osmolality. **(M-S)**

Hypnosis is used to treat psychogenic amnesia. **(PSY)**

Hypertension is a sign of rejection of a transplanted kidney. **(M-S)**

Lactulose is used to prevent and treat portal-systemic encephalopathy. **(M-S)**

A child's failure to grow above the third percentile in 2 years may be related to hypopituitarism. **(PED)**

Extracorporeal and intracorporeal shock wave lithotripsy is the use of shock waves to perform noninvasive destruction of biliary stones. It's indicated in the treatment of symptomatic high-risk patients who have few noncalcified cholesterol stones. **(M-S)**

Disulfiram (Antabuse) is administered orally as an aversion therapy to treat alcoholism. **(PSY)**

Ingestion of alcohol by a patient who is taking disulfiram (Antabuse) can cause severe reactions, including nausea and vomiting, and may endanger the patient's life. **(PSY)**

Clinical manifestations of congenital dislocation of the hip include gluteal folds, with deeper creases apparent on the affected side, and limited hip abduction on the affected side which produces a click (Ortolani's click). **(PED)**

Cretinism is suspected when the mother reports that her baby sleeps all the time and doesn't cry. He may even be described as a "good baby." **(PED)**

Decreased consciousness is a clinical sign of an increased ammonia level in a patient with kidney failure or cirrhosis of the liver. **(M-S)**

The pain medication that's given to patients who have acute pancreatitis is meperidine (Demerol). **(M-S)**

Prochlorperazine (Compazine), meclizine, and trimethobenzamide (Tigan) are used to treat the nausea and vomiting caused by cholecystitis. **(M-S)**

▓ Improved concentration is a sign that lithium is taking effect. **(PSY)**

▓ Behavior modification, including time-outs, token economy, or a reward system, is a treatment for attention deficit hyperactivity disorder. **(PSY)**

▓ Obese women are more susceptible to gallstones than any other group. **(M-S)**

▓ Metabolic acidosis is a common finding in acute renal failure. **(M-S)**

▓ For a patient who has anorexia nervosa, the nurse should provide support at mealtime and record the amount the patient eats. **(PSY)**

▓ For a patient who has acute pancreatitis, the most important nursing intervention is to maintain his fluid and electrolyte balance. **(M-S)**

▓ After thyroidectomy, the patient is monitored for hypocalcemia. **(M-S)**

▓ In end-stage cirrhosis of the liver, the patient's ammonia level is elevated. **(M-S)**

▓ In a patient who has liver cirrhosis, abdominal girth is measured with the superior iliac crest used as a landmark. **(M-S)**

▓ *Biliary atresia* is congenital absence or underdevelopment of one or more of the biliary structures. It causes jaundice and early liver damage. As the condition worsens, the child's growth may be retarded and portal hypertension may develop. **(PED)**

▓ The symptoms of Alzheimer's disease have an insidious onset. **(M-S)**

▓ A significant toxic risk associated with clozapine (Clozaril) administration is blood dyscrasia. **(PSY)**

▓ Fracture of the skull in the area of the cerebellum may cause ataxia and inability to coordinate movement. **(M-S)**

▓ The nurse should use time-outs to help control the behavior of the hyperactive child. **(PED)**

▓ Adverse effects of haloperidol (Haldol) administration include drowsiness; insomnia; weakness; headache; and extrapyramidal symptoms, such as akathisia, tardive dyskinesia, and dystonia. **(PSY)**

▓ Serum creatinine is the laboratory test that provides the most specific indication of kidney disease. **(M-S)**

A patient who has bilateral adrenalectomy must take cortisone for the rest of his life. (M-S)

Hypervigilance and déjà vu are signs of posttraumatic stress disorder (PTSD). (PSY)

Portal vein hypertension causes esophageal varices. (M-S)

A symptom of childhood-onset autism is the inability to focus because of impulsiveness and inattention. (PED)

A child who shows dissociation has probably been abused. (PSY)

Signs and symptoms of hypoxia include tachycardia, shortness of breath, cyanosis, and mottled skin. (M-S)

A child who has galactosemia shouldn't be given milk products. (PED)

Failure to thrive is usually associated with a heart defect. (PED)

Collegiality is the promotion of collaboration, development, and inter-dependence among members of a profession. (FND)

A *change agent* is an individual who recognizes a need for change or is se-lected to make a change within an established entity, such as a hospital. (FND)

The passage of normal brown feces usually indicates that intussuscep-tion, or telescoping of a segment of the colon, has corrected itself. (PED)

In a child, a urinary tract infection causes incontinence (in a toilet-trained child), strong-smelling urine, and urinary frequency or urgency. (PED)

If the nurse notices that a girl or woman has been circumcised, she must be careful to avoid showing disgust or surprise but should discuss her observation with the patient or with the parent, if the patient is a child. (PED)

To prevent oral burns in the infant, breast milk shouldn't be thawed or rewarmed in a microwave oven. (PED)

Strict isolation is required for children who have chickenpox or diph-theria. (PED)

■ The three types of embolism are air, fat, and thrombus. (M-S)

■ The patients' bill of rights was introduced by the American Hospital Association. (FND)

■ *Abandonment* is premature termination of treatment without the patient's permission and without appropriate relief of symptoms. (FND)

■ Associations for patients who have had laryngeal cancer include the Lost Cord Club and the New Voice Club. (M-S)

■ Before discharge, a patient who has had a total laryngectomy must be able to perform tracheostomy care and suctioning and use alternative means of communication. (M-S)

■ The universal blood donor is O negative. (M-S)

■ The universal blood recipient is AB positive. (M-S)

■ Mucus in a colostomy bag indicates that the colon is beginning to function. (M-S)

■ After a vasectomy, the patient is considered sterile if he has no sperm cells. (M-S)

■ Fatigue is an adverse effect of radiation therapy. (M-S)

■ The child who has celiac disease may eat rice. (PED)

■ To prevent dumping syndrome, the patient's consumption of high-carbohydrate foods and liquids should be limited. (M-S)

■ Pelvic-tilt exercises can help to prevent or relieve backache during pregnancy. (MAT)

■ *Confabulation* is the use of fantasy to fill in gaps of memory. (PSY)

■ *Values clarification* is a process that individuals use to prioritize their personal values. (FND)

■ *Distributive justice* is a principle that promotes equal treatment for all. (FND)

■ Before performing a Leopold maneuver, the nurse should ask the patient to empty her bladder. (MAT)

▦ Milk and milk products, poultry, grains, and fish are good sources of phosphate. **(FND)**

▦ Cryoprecipitate contains factors VIII and XIII and fibrinogen and is used to treat hemophilia. **(M-S)**

▦ Insomnia is the most common sleep disorder. **(M-S)**

▦ *Bruxism* is grinding of the teeth during sleep. **(M-S)**

▦ The best way to prevent falls at night in an oriented, but restless, elderly patient is to raise the side rails. **(FND)**

▦ By the end of the orientation phase, the patient should begin to trust the nurse. **(FND)**

▦ Listening is the most effective communication technique to use with a child who stutters. **(PED)**

▦ Falls in the elderly are likely to be caused by poor vision. **(FND)**

▦ Barriers to communication include language deficits, sensory deficits, cognitive impairments, structural deficits, and paralysis. **(FND)**

▦ The three elements that are necessary for a fire are heat, oxygen, and combustible material. **(FND)**

▦ Sebaceous glands lubricate the skin. **(FND)**

▦ Elderly patients are at risk for osteoporosis because of age-related bone demineralization. **(M-S)**

▦ To check for petechiae in a dark-skinned patient, the nurse should assess the oral mucosa. **(FND)**

▦ The clinical manifestations of local infection in an extremity are tenderness, loss of use of the extremity, erythema, edema, and warmth. **(M-S)**

▦ Clinical manifestations of systemic infection include fever and swollen lymph nodes. **(M-S)**

▦ To put on a sterile glove, the nurse should pick up the first glove at the folded border and adjust the fingers when both gloves are on. **(FND)**

▦ An immobile patient is predisposed to thrombus formation because of increased blood stasis. **(M-S)**

- To increase patient comfort, the nurse should let the alcohol dry before giving an intramuscular injection.   (FND)

- Treatment for a stage 1 ulcer on the heels includes heel protectors.
                                                                          (FND)

- Seventh-Day Adventists are usually vegetarians.   (FND)

- Urea is the chief end product of amino acid metabolism.   (M-S)

- Morphine and other opioids relieve pain by binding to the nerve cells in the dorsal horn of the spinal cord.   (M-S)

- Endorphins are morphinelike substances that produce a feeling of well-being.   (FND)

- *Pain tolerance* is the maximum amount and duration of pain that an individual is willing to endure.   (FND)

- *Trichomonas* and *Candida* infections can be acquired nonsexually. (M-S)

- *Presbycusis* is progressive sensorineural hearing loss that occurs as part of the aging process.   (M-S)

Index

A

Abandonment, 224
ABCDE cascade, 199
Abdominal assessment, 196
Abdominal distention, 138, 214
Abdominal pain, 76, 111. *See also* Pain.
ABO blood groups, 56, 224
Abortion, 28, 46, 112, 130
Abruptio placentae, 37, 42, 74
Abuse, 193, 220. *See also* *specific type.*
Accessory muscle use, 83
Accidents, children and, 79
ACE inhibitors, 152, 198
Acetaminophen overdose, 62
Acid-base balance, 13, 55, 93, 176
Acid perfusion test, 113
Acne, 217
Acquired immunodeficiency syndrome, 18, 55, 60, 145, 168. *See also* Human immunodeficiency virus infection.
Acrocyanosis, 142
Active assistance exercises, 136
Activities of daily living, 85, 135

Acute alcohol withdrawal, 120-121
Acute tubular necrosis, 90
Addisonian crisis, 86
Addison's disease, 10
Adhesions, 126
Adolescent, eating habits of, 133
Adrenalectomy, 54, 223
Adult respiratory distress syndrome, 70
Afterload, 35, 164
Against medical advice, 115
Agoraphobia, 218
AIDS, 18, 55, 60, 145, 168. *See also* HIV infection.
Airway, removing, 8
Airway obstruction, 135, 193
Airway patency, maintaining, 32, 66
Alanine aminotransferase levels, 95
Al-Anon, 5, 218
Albumin, 177
Alcohol, metabolism of, 25, 69
Alcoholic
   life stresses and, 45
   recovering, 5
   therapeutic regimen for, 72
   thiamine therapy for, 139

Alcoholic beverage, proof of, 69
Alcoholics Anonymous, 38, 65
Alcoholism, 139
Alcohol withdrawal, 5, 71, 72, 139
Aldosterone, 201
Allergen, 125
allopurinol (Zyloprim), 19
Alpha-fetoprotein, 22, 157, 207
aluminum hydroxide (Amphojel), 18, 55, 63
Alzheimer's disease, 23, 60, 90, 116, 222
Ambulation, 32-33, 67, 202
Amenorrhea, 6, 97
Aminoglycosides, 137
aminophylline (Aminophyllin), 150
amitriptyline (Elavil), 191
Ammonia, sources of, 181
Amnesia, 49, 221
Amniocentesis, 45, 121, 205
Amniotomy, 5
Amputation, 16, 36, 60, 74, 90, 100, 119, 123, 143, 167
Amyotrophic lateral sclerosis, 56
Analgesics, 216
Anaphylaxis, 81

227

Anemia, 179. *See also specific type.*
Anesthesia, 65, 66, 67, 205
Anesthetics, 80, 109
Angina, 41, 113, 115, 162, 163, 198
Angiography, 16
Angioplasty, 135
Angiotensin-converting enzyme inhibitors, 152, 198
Angry patient, 66, 78, 141
Anisocoria, 175
Anorexia nervosa, 4, 38, 145, 178, 222
Antacids, 158
Antiarrhythmic agents, 198
Antibiotics, 137, 172, 175
Anticholinergic drugs, 184
Anticholinesterase agents, 99
Anticoagulants, 7, 28, 44, 209
Antidiabetic agents, 120, 192
Antiembolism stockings, 54, 163-164. *See also* Elastic stockings.
Antihistamines, 21
Antihypertensive drugs, 199
Antisocial personality disorder, 89
Anuria, 3
Anxiety, 4, 66, 118
Aortic aneurysm, 159
Aortic dissection, 152
Aortic stenosis, 73
Apgar score, 9, 139
Apnea, 78
Appendicitis, 22, 76, 138
Arm fracture, 128
Arrhythmias, 51, 152, 198, 215
Arterial blood, 80
Arterial blood gas analysis, 113
Arterial disease, 153
Arterial embolism, 102
Arthritis, 63
Arthrography, 63

Artificial eye, caring for, 106
Ascites, 25, 50, 138, 141, 181, 217
asparaginase, 51
Aspartate aminotransferase levels, 95
aspirin, 158
aspirin toxicity, 84, 105
Assault, 118. *See also* Battery *and* Sexual assault.
Assessment data, collecting, 15, 30, 46, 71, 78, 94, 103, 116, 168, 189, 196
Asthma, 46, 54, 97, 107, 134, 152, 169, 202, 208
Ataxia, 115, 190
Ataxic gait, 94
Atelectasis, 52, 178, 202. *See also* Postoperative complications.
Atherosclerosis, 100, 117
Atrioventricular valves, 104
atropine, 85, 95, 98, 110
Attention deficit hyperactivity disorder, 65, 91, 220, 222
Autism, 46, 50, 223
Autonomic nervous system, 62, 99
Autotransfusion, 102

B

Babinski's reflex, 53, 148
Back pain, 187
baclofen (Lioresal), 166
Bagging as ventilatory method, 17
Ballottement, 105
Barbiturate coma, 76
Barbiturates, 63
Barium enema, 214
Basal cell carcinoma, 169, 202
Basal metabolic rate, 24
Battery, 168. *See also* Assault.
Battle's sign, 136
Bed bath, 63

Bedside care, 11
Bell's palsy, 29, 128
Bence Jones protein, 96
Beneficence, 199
Benign prostatic hyperplasia, 37
Benign tumors, 174
benztropine (Cogentin), 219
Beriberi, 31
Beta-adrenergic blockers, 162
Biliary atresia, 222
Bipolar affective disorder, 60, 65, 190, 216
bisacodyl, 158
Bivalve cast, 106
Bladder aspiration, 20, 33
Bladder carcinoma, 6
Bladder distention, 13, 40, 53, 106
Bladder infection, 69
Bladder irrigation, 106, 107
Bladder retraining, 61, 213
Bland diet, 136
Blindness, 84
Blood alcohol level, determining, 194
Blood and body fluids, handling, 96, 149
Blood clot, dislodging, 109
Blood cultures, 152
Blood glucose level, 124, 125, 156, 210, 218
Blood loss, 36, 80
Blood pH, 113
Blood pressure, 39, 111, 118
   measuring, 2, 3, 39, 40, 79, 109, 161, 197
   orthostatic, 80
Blood transfusion, 7, 22, 30, 101, 102, 123, 132, 133, 180
Blood urea nitrogen, 88, 202, 188
Body alignment, 111
Body temperature, 107
   factors that affect, 103
   measuring, 31, 47, 130
Bone age, determining, 197

Bone cancer, 195
Bone healing, 98
Bone infection, 59
Bone marrow, 35
Bone marrow aspiration, 26, 57, 180
Bone marrow transplantation, 210
Bone pain, 85
Borderline personality disorder, 49, 65
Bottle-feeding, 149, 156, 197, 208
Botulism, 30
Bowel obstruction, 44, 96, 132, 150
Bowel sounds, 190
Bradford frame, 19, 24
Bradycardia, 102
Bradykinesia, 177
Brain, 142
Brain attack. See Stroke.
Brain damage, 9, 53, 95, 146
Brain death, 21, 200
Brain surgery, 53, 54, 165, 188
Brain tumors, 213
Braxton Hicks contractions, 76
Breast cancer, 36, 169, 207
Breast-feeding, 2, 29, 33, 48, 53, 70, 93, 147, 149, 155-156, 191, 193, 209, 210, 211, 223
Breast self-examination, 153, 206
Breath sounds, 67
Breech birth, 68
Brompton's cocktail, 63
Bronchodilators, 201
Bronchopulmonary dysplasia, 196
Bronchoscopy, 189
Brudzinski's sign, 166
Bruits, 82, 105
Bruxism, 225
Bryant's traction, 2
Buck's traction, 118, 128
Bulimia, 145

buprenorphine (Buprenex), 216
Burn injury, 97, 107, 185, 214
Burn patient
    bathing, 110
    black feces in, 184
    care priorities for, 7, 118, 184
    hospitalizing, 58
    hyperkalemia in, 184
    infection and, 117
    leading cause of death of, 6, 187
    nutritional needs of, 186
    physiologic changes in, 59
    skin graft and, 184
    wound care for, 11, 110
Butterfly rash, 26

C
calcifediol (Calderol), 88
Calcium channel blockers, 162, 198
Calcium, 95
Caloric intake, 215
Cancer, 63, 88, 120, 181. See also specific type.
Candidiasis, 19, 89, 179, 185, 193, 226
Cane walking, 13, 30, 179
Capillary refill, 15
captopril (Capoten), 152
Caput succedaneum, 148
Carbon dioxide, arterial, partial pressure of, 114
Carbon monoxide poisoning, 59, 213
Cardiac arrest, 2, 5
Cardiac catheterization, 25, 97, 139, 159-160, 179, 207, 212
Cardiac glycosides, 17, 170, 198, 208, 215
Cardiac output, 80, 81, 140, 142, 159
Cardiac surgery, 120
Cardiac tamponade, 191
Cardinal fields of gaze, 137

Cardiogenic shock, 50, 77, 85
Cardiopulmonary bypass graft, 111
Cardiopulmonary resuscitation, 52, 76, 114, 135
Cardioversion, 114
Carminative enema, 214
Carpal tunnel syndrome, 129, 196
Cast care, 186, 188
Casts, 118, 128
Cataract, 127, 137, 204
Cataract removal, 68, 106
Catharsis, 98
Catheterization, 24
Celiac disease, 46, 150, 224
Cellulitis, 134
Central venous catheters, 130
Central venous pressure, 43, 80, 161, 207
Cephalosporins, 112, 137
Cerebral palsy, 68, 90, 186
Cerebrospinal fluid, 94, 123, 175
Cerebrovascular accident. See Stroke.
Cervical cancer, 25, 36, 61, 120, 178, 206
Cervical injury, 166
Cervical ripening, 147, 211
Cervical secretions, 91
Cervical suturing, 93
Cesarean birth, 67, 121, 157, 184
Chalazion, 137
Chancre, 23
Change agent, 223
Cheilosis, 24, 214
Chemotherapy, 52, 110, 149, 169, 212
Chest drainage system, 6, 37, 74, 78, 101, 102, 139
Chest excursion, 83
Chest pain, 13, 41, 100, 118, 159, 162, 195, 212

Chest physiotherapy, 86, 191. *See also* Postural drainage.
Chest surgery, 88
Chest tube, 52, 102, 153
Cheyne-Stokes respirations, 78
Chickenpox, 7, 69, 17, 2239
Child
administering medication to, 21, 80, 171
communicating with, 20, 78, 86, 150, 188
diet for, 136
dying, 44-45, 211
growth failure and, 221
hospitalized, 42, 166
normal behaviors in, 19
offering choices to, 192
poor appetite in, 20
rating pain in, 204
taking temperature of, 47
teaching, about postoperative events, 31
water temperature for, 34
Child abuse, 19, 43, 97, 168, 183, 223
Child neglect, 89
Chlamydial infection, 83, 145
Chloasma, 14, 154
chloral hydrate suppositories, 128
chloramphenicol, 113
chlordiazepoxide (Librium), 71
chlorpromazine (Thorazine), 5, 18
chlorpropamide (Diabinese), 120
Choking, universal sign of, 5
Cholecystectomy, 178
Cholecystitis, 95, 138, 220, 221
Cholecystography, 63, 64
Cholelithiasis, 55, 62
Cholesterol, 34, 159
Cholesterol test, 113
cholestyramine (Questran), 211

Chorea, 194
Chorion, 46
Chorionic villus sampling, 155
Chromosomes, 23, 196
Chronic obstructive pulmonary disease, 21, 134, 142
cimetidine (Tagamet), 119, 123
Circulatory disturbances, 129
Circumcision, 156, 223
Circumstantiality as thought disturbance, 81
Cirrhosis, 62, 117, 122, 132, 217, 219, 220, 221, 222
Clark's rule, pediatric dose calculation and, 7
Cleft lip or palate, 49, 73, 83
Climacteric, 53
clindamycin, 150
clomiphene (Clomid), 93
clozapine (Clozaril), 220, 222
colchicine (Colsalide), 97, 182
Cold application, 97, 99
Collaboration, 102, 133
Collegiality, 223
Colonic irrigation, 133, 143
Colorectal cancer, 23, 126, 212
Colostomy, 49, 51, 52, 54, 58, 77, 84, 89, 102, 143, 149, 224
Colostomy care, 10, 210
Colostrum, 59
Comatose patient, 61
Comfort measures, 32
Communication, 171, 172, 182, 190, 192, 194, 202, 216, 225
Compartmental syndrome, 166
Compulsion, 26
Conduct disorder, 193
Confabulation, 66, 224

Confrontation as communication technique, 121
Congenital heart defects, 122, 189, 190, 192, 223. *See also specific defect.*
Congenital megacolon, 38
Consent for treatment, 8
Constipation, 18, 104, 119
Contraception, 34
Contraceptives, 40-41, 46, 100, 130
Contractures, 99
Controlled substances, 116, 132-133
Conversion disorder, 68
COPD, 21, 134, 142
Corneal injury, 106
Cornea transplantation, 45, 68, 127
Coronary artery bypass grafting, 33, 161-162
Coronary artery disease, 79, 100, 114, 161
Corpus luteum, 46
Cow's milk, 13
CPR, 52, 76, 114, 135
Crackles, 136, 178, 198
Cranial nerves, 94, 175
Craniotomy, 86, 188
Creatine kinase-MB, 2, 27, 77, 163
Creatinine, 222
Creatinine clearance, 202
Creative intuition, 64
Cretinism, 221
Crisis intervention, 190
Critical pathways, 169
Crohn's disease, 72, 185
Croup, 43, 198
Crowning, 135, 155
Crutches, 13, 40
Crutch walking, 30-31, 84, 126-127, 172
Cryoprecipitate, 225
Culdoscopy, 77
Cullen's sign, 32
Cultural customs, 194, 216
Cushing's syndrome, 86, 217
Cutis marmorata, 37

Cyanosis, 11, 32
cyclosporine (Sandimmune), 70
Cystic fibrosis, 57, 60, 89, 134
Cystourethrography, 82
Cytomegalovirus infection, 70, 89, 119

D

Death and dying, 45, 119
  child and, 44-45, 68
  five stages of, 2
Debridement, 106, 171, 183
Decibel, 8, 57
Decorticate posturing, 122
Deep vein thrombosis, 43, 100, 189
Defense mechanisms, 47
Defibrillation, 197
Dehiscence, 85, 165, 192
Dehydration, 42, 54, 64, 84, 106, 177, 214
Delivery
  emergency, 60
  mechanics of, 96
  pelvic measurements and, 59, 203
  pelvis types and, 14
  umbilical cord and, 9
Delusions, 216, 218
Dementia, 189
Denial, 13, 76, 219
Dentures, cleaning, 61
Dependent behavior, 65
Depression, 10, 65, 66, 74, 89, 181, 190, 196
Desensitization, 26, 177, 218
Detoxification, 72
Developmental stages, 7, 12, 28, 36, 38, 47, 49, 77, 79, 80, 91, 115, 120, 182, 192, 199
dexamethasone (Decadron), 167, 213
Diabetes insipidus, 64, 87, 217, 221

Diabetes mellitus, 84, 117, 124, 125, 173, 204, 205, 218, 220
Diabetic coma, 87
Diabetic neuropathy, 218
Dialysis, 17, 20, 21, 60, 178. *See also specific type.*
Diaper, determining urine content of, 185
Diarrhea, 20, 195
Dick test, 58
Dietary fiber, 25
Diffusion, 72
Digestion, 94, 176
digoxin (Lanoxin), 7, 17, 115, 158, 185, 209
digoxin toxicity, 2, 7, 53, 88, 198, 202, 215
Dilatation and curettage, 130
diltiazem (Cardizem), 111, 162
diphenhydramine (Benadryl), 64
Diphtheria, 223
Direct antiglobulin test, 122
Direct Coombs' test, 122
Disability, 100
Discrimination, 194
Disequilibrium syndrome, 56
Disk, ruptured, 186
Displacement of unacceptable feelings, 76
Distributive justice, 224
Disulfiram (Antabuse), 48, 49, 138, 221
Diuretics, 152, 158, 188, 215
Diverticulitis, 185
Documentation, 71, 103, 107
Docusate (Colace), 120
Doll's eye movement, 156
Double-bind communication, 157
Down syndrome, 43, 146, 156, 157, 203
Drainage on dressing, 51, 89

Dressler's syndrome, 164
Drug absorption, 195
Drug action, 93
Drug names, 35
Drug overdose, 66
Drug toxicity, 66
Dumping syndrome, 56, 146, 224
Dyspnea, 72, 214

E

Ear examination, 49
Ear irrigation, 67, 106
Ear medication, 171
Ear wax, 129
ECG, 77, 115, 198
Echocardiography, 115
Echolalia, 11
Eclampsia, 42, 138
Ectoderm, 46
Ectopic pregnancy, 27, 95
Edema, 38, 92, 150, 165, 177, 181
Egalitarian theory, 200
Ego, 11
Elastic stockings, 7, 140. *See also* Antiembolism stockings.
Elder abuse, 119
Elective surgery, 73
Electrocardiography, 77, 115, 198
Electroconvulsive therapy, 51, 56-57, 64, 195, 218, 219, 220
Electroencephalography, 61
Electrolyte imbalance, 181, 195, 215
Electrolytes, measuring, in solution, 24
Emancipated minor, 8
Embolism, 163, 224. *See also specific type.*
Embryo, 197
Emergency surgery, 73
Emotional development, 18
Emphysema, 21, 208
enalapril (Vasotec), 152
Endorphins, 226
Endoscopy, 208
Enemas, 109, 177, 213, 214

Engagement, fetal descent and, 9
Enteric feeding, 214
Enteric precautions, 64
Epididymitis, 22, 150
Epigastric pain, 91
Epiglottiditis, 76, 167, 183, 198
epinephrine (Adrenalin), 2, 62, 75, 143
Epistaxis, 111
ergotamine (Ergomar), 62
Eruption of teeth, 74, 150
Erythroblastosis fetalis, 74
Erythrocyte sedimentation rate, 77, 113
erythromycin, 50, 101, 150, 213
Erythropoiesis, 178, 213
Esophageal balloon tamponade, 6, 179
Esophageal cancer, 212
Esophageal varices, 44, 180, 219, 223
Estriol levels, 169
Estrogen replacement therapy, 87
Ethnocentrism, 194
Eupnea, 79
Euthanasia, 200, 201
Evaluation as nursing process step, 16, 71, 105
Exchange transfusions, 101
Excretory urography, 108, 217
Exercise ECG, 114, 162
Exercise stress test. See Exercise ECG.
Expiratory grunting, 156
Extramural delivery, 212
Extrapyramidal reactions, 64, 66, 184, 219
Extravasation, 169
Eye care, 144
Eye examination, 105, 109, 137
Eye injury, 126
Eye irrigation, 106
Eye medications, 58, 68, 171
Eye patch, 126, 127

Eye surgery, 45, 109, 126, 127, 204

F
Family coping, 153, 184, 194
Family therapy, 77
Farsightedness, 126
Fasting blood glucose level, 2, 18
Fasting plasma glucose test, 113
Fat embolism, 3, 61, 74
Fat emulsion, 23
Fear, 66
Fecal impaction, 201
Fecal occult blood test, 119, 213
Femoral-popliteal bypass graft, 54-55
Femur fracture, 4, 39, 185
Fertility, 205
Fertilization, 35, 98, 196
Fetal alcohol syndrome, 17, 155
Fetal demise, 119
Fetal embodiment, 153
Fetal heart rate, 17, 29
Fetal monitoring, 16, 59, 88, 92
Fetal station, 9
Fetal well-being, assessing, 91
Fetus, 46
Fever, 3, 54, 127, 190, 193, 214
Fibrocystic breast disease, 189
Fight-or-flight response, 66
Fire, 10, 225
Flail chest, 207
flavoxate (Urispas), 50
Flight of ideas, 4, 192
Floating, fetal descent and, 9
Fluid and electrolyte balance, 108, 177, 181, 193, 213, 214
Fluid overload, 180
Fluid retention, 79
Fluorescein staining, 22

Fluorescent treponemal antibody absorption test, 127
Fluoride treatment, 68
fluoxetine (Prozac), 110, 194
flurazepam (Dalmane), 89
Folic acid, 86, 92, 121, 203
Folic acid deficiency, 214
Fontanel, 4, 147
Food diary, 213
Food poisoning, 142
Foot cradle, 105
Footdrop, 8, 74
Foreign body removal from eye, 106
Fractures, 69, 98, 119, 183. See also specific type.
Frostbite, 105
F/TPAL system, 154
Fugue, 148
Fundal height, 12, 27, 189, 203, 205
Fungal infections, 131. See also specific type.
furosemide (Lasix), 158, 201, 202, 205, 215

G
Gait, 85
Galactorrhea, 6
Galactosemia, 223
Gallbladder removal, 220
Gangrene, 39, 151
Gastrectomy, 51, 138, 146
Gastric lavage, 51, 105
Gastric suctioning, 213
Gastric surgery, 51
Gastric ulcer, 4, 11, 53, 94, 110, 135, 136
Gastroenteritis, 142
Gastroesophageal reflux, 67
Gastrointestinal bleeding, 110, 181
Gastrostomy feeding, 214
Gaucher's disease, 96
Gauge of needle, 107
Gavage, 3
Gender identity, 145, 219
General adaptation syndrome, 171

Geriatric patient, 23, 80, 88, 97, 103-104, 133, 141, 172-173, 205, 225
Gestational age, 139
Glasgow Coma Scale, 122, 175
Glaucoma, 10, 84, 98, 182, 185, 203, 204, 205, 206
Glomerulonephritis, 190, 195
Gloves, sterile, 225
Glucocorticoid therapy, 211, 215
Glucose-6-phospate dehydrogenase deficiency, 8, 26, 93
Glucose tolerance test, 220
Gonorrhea, 8, 38, 50, 143, 184
Goodell's sign, 12
Good Samaritan laws, 115
Gout, 97, 104, 182
Gouty arthritis, 118
Graft-versus-host reaction, 180
Graves' disease, 69, 117
Gravida, definition of, 27
Grieving, 26, 64
griseofulvin (Grisovin FP), 158
Group therapy, 87
Growth disturbances, 60
Guillain-Barré syndrome, 19, 22, 188
Guthrie test, 149
Gynecomastia, 116, 210

H

Habitual aborter, 28
Hair care, 144
Hair removal for surgery, 111
haloperidol (Haldol), 222
Handheld resuscitation bag, 102, 150
Hand washing, 23
Harlequin sign, 148
Harris flush, 214
Head injury, 61
Head lice, 184-185

Health care, 216
Health history, 103
Health records, 116
Healthy People 2010, 205
Hearing, 55, 57, 67, 185, 206, 226
Hearing aid, 67, 144, 173
Hearing-impaired patient, 127, 171, 182
Heart, 118
Heart failure, 5, 33, 52, 53, 84, 87, 118, 150, 152, 163, 164, 165, 198, 208
Heart murmurs, 138, 159
Heart sounds, 118, 159, 190
Heat application, 112
Heat exhaustion, 129
Heatstroke, 129
Hegar's sign, 12
HELLP syndrome, 157
Hemagglutination inhibition test, 9
Hemangiomas, 148
Hemianopsia, 56, 176, 188
Hemoccult test, 119, 213
Hemodialysis, 39, 41
Hemoglobin, 209
Hemoglobin electrophoresis test, 150
Hemolysis, 81
Hemophilia, 25
Hemorrhage, 122, 181
Hemorrhagic shock, 15
Hemorrhoids, 110
Heparin, 6, 10, 17, 43, 144, 178, 209
Heparin lock, 70, 113
Hepatic encephalopathy, 217
Hepatitis, 60, 64, 140, 185. *See also specific type.*
Hepatitis A, 6, 63, 64, 219
Hepatitis B, 72, 112, 124
Hepatitis B immune globulin,112, 157
Hepatitis B vaccine, 39, 51, 157
Hepatitis C, 167, 181
Hernia, 62, 64, 137, 152, 187

Herniated disk, 4
Heroin withdrawal in neonate, 17
Herpes simplex infection, 82
Herpes zoster, 179, 187
Hertz, 57
Hiccups, postoperative, 49
High-carbohydrate foods, 146, 172
High-fiber diet, 25, 143
High-potassium diet, 78
Hip dislocation, 183, 221
Hip dysplasia, 49
Hip fracture, 15, 118, 128
Hip nailing, preventing external rotation after, 11
Hip prosthesis, hip pain and, 11
Hip replacement, 186
Hirschsprung's disease, 38
Hirsutism, 132
Histoplasmosis, 6
HIV infection, 26, 53, 96, 179. *See also* AIDS.
Hodgkin's disease, 11, 25, 28, 90
Homans' sign, 24, 109
Hordeolum, 137
Hormone therapy, 217
Hot flash, 24
Hoyer lift, 129
Human chorionic gonadotropin, 98, 122, 206
Human immunodeficiency virus infection, 26, 53, 96, 179. *See also* Acquired immunodeficiency syndrome.
Human personality, levels of, 46
Humidity in room, 23
Huntington's disease, 90
Hyaline membrane disease, 20
Hydramnios, 28
Hydrocephalus, 190, 194
Hyperaldosteronism, 19
Hypercalcemia, 195
Hyperemesis gravidarum, 151

Hyperglycemia, 117
Hyperinsulinism, 91
Hyperkalemia, 184, 218
Hypernatremia, 213
Hyperopia, 99
Hyperparathyroidism, 195
Hyperpigmentation, 154
Hyperproteinemia, 217
Hyperpyrexia, 190
Hypertension, 205
Hypertensive crisis, 169, 208, 219
Hyperthyroidism, 69, 151. *See also* Graves' disease.
Hypertonic solutions, 103
Hyperuricemia, 97
Hyperventilation, 78, 98, 194
Hypervolemia, 188
Hypocalcemia, 6, 123
Hypochondriasis, 76
Hypoglycemia, 83, 125, 180
Hypokalemia, 2, 30, 140
Hyponatremia, 92, 214
Hypoparathyroidism, 219
Hypopituitarism, 146, 221
Hypospadias, 156
Hypotension, 141
Hypothalamus, 83, 142
Hypothermia, 146
Hypothyroidism, 133, 217
Hypotonic enema, 213
Hypotonic solutions, 103
Hypoventilation, 211
Hypovolemia, 33, 57, 214
Hypovolemic shock, 56
Hypoxemia, 178
Hypoxia, 213, 223
Hysterectomy, 36

I

Ice water lavage, 90
Id, 12
Idea of reference in psychiatry, 84
Identification band, 3, 129, 143, 212
Ileal conduit, 52, 74
Ileostomy, 49, 54, 91, 108

Ileus
  mechanical, 50
  paralytic, 21
Illness, 216
Illusion, 65
I.M. injection, 60, 144, 168, 226. *See also* Z-track I.M. injection.
imipramine (Tofranil), 217
Immunization, 7, 51, 75, 135, 187, 204, 212
Immunosuppressants, 128
Immunosuppression, 70
Imperforate anus, 89
Impetigo, 135, 187
Implementation as nursing process step, 16, 71
Incentive spirometry, 32, 37
Incident report, 168
Incontinence, 40. *See also specific type.*
Individual coping, 206
Indwelling catheter, 106
Infancy period, 47
Infant
  administering medication to, 20, 147, 197
  dehydration in, 42, 106, 156
  diabetic mother and, 139, 183
  diaper changing and, 29
  diarrhea in, 20
  Down syndrome in, 43
  examining ear of, 49
  exposure of, 146
  feeding, through tracheostomy tube, 29
  gastrostomy tube and, 83
  hospitalized, transporting, 42
  human immunodeficiency virus and, 96
  I.V. therapy for, 80
  lifting, 34
  maternal separation and, 19
  monitoring growth and development of, 47, 55, 66

Infant *(continued)*
  nasotracheal suctioning in, 26
  scalp vein infusion in, 34
  sleeping position for, 20
  solid food for, 20, 156, 195
  tooth eruption in, 74
  vital signs, 198
  weight gain in, 36, 55
Infection, 35, 87, 173, 181, 225
Inferior vena cava syndrome, 150
Inflammatory response, 171
Informed consent, 8, 74, 78, 104, 173
Inhalation therapy, 193
Inheritance patterns, 201
Injections, 20, 144, 151. *See also specific type.*
Insomnia, 225
Inspection as assessment technique, 79
Insulin, 124
Insulin deficiency, 117
Insulin therapy, 3, 15, 105, 108, 124, 125, 139
Intermittent claudication, 6, 33
Intermittent positive-pressure breathing, 7, 99
Intestinal obstruction, 44
Intracellular fluid, 30
Intracranial bleeding, 93
Intracranial pressure, 88
Intracranial pressure, increased, 4, 11, 61, 76, 167, 180, 183, 190
Intracranial surgery, 86
Intradermal injection, 109, 197
Intraocular pressure, 15, 88, 182. *See also* Glaucoma.
Intraoperative period, 31
Intraperitoneal shunt, 176
Intrathecal injection, 202
Intussusception, 96, 223
Ipecac syrup, 45, 15, 1861
Iridectomy, 204

Iron, sources of, 101, 201
Iron deficiency anemia, 14
Iron supplements, 35, 151, 155, 158, 196
Ischemia, 163
isoetharine (Bronkosol), 21
Isolation precautions, 58, 59, 117, 131, 149, 175
Isometric exercises, 135, 173
isoniazid, 158
Isotonic solutions, 103
I.V. antibiotics, 119
I.V. cholangiography, 117
I.V. push, 29
I.V. solutions, 103
I.V. therapy, 80, 101, 129, 130, 131, 133, 168

J

Jackson-Pratt drainage system, 170
Jaundice, 13, 74, 92, 109, 123, 219
Jehovah's witnesses, 22
Jugular vein distention, 84

K

Kaposi's sarcoma, 154, 179
Kawasaki disease, 86
Kegel exercises, 141, 204
Keloid, 145
Keratitis, 128
Kernig's sign, 4, 166
Ketoacidosis, 57, 125, 207
Ketones, 18, 220
Kidney cancer, 209
Kidney function, 39, 202
Kidneys, 120
Kidney transplantation, 36, 41
Kilocalorie, 69
Knee replacement, 56, 175
Knowledge, assessing level of, 193
Koplik's spots, 12
Korsakoff's syndrome, 88, 139, 140
Kussmaul's respirations, 78, 143, 207
Kyphosis, 177

L

La belle indifference, 4
Labile affect, 49
Labor
    cervical dilation and, 29
    clinical features of, 2
    contractions in, 13, 14, 15, 29, 57, 155
    fetal descent in, 9, 157
    fetal heart rate and, 120
    fetal heart tones in, 69, 131
    hypotension during, 92
    inducing, 119
    precipitate, 75
    premature rupture of membranes and, 178, 192
    side-lying position in, 9, 83, 195
    spinal block in, 92
    stages of, 27, 207
Laboratory test results, 103
Lactulose, 221
Ladin's sign, 154
Laminaria, 211
Laminectomy, 4, 196
Lanugo, 83
Laryngeal cancer, 87, 224
Laryngectomy, 209, 224
Laryngotracheobronchitis, 211
Lead poisoning, 19, 84, 187, 203
Leg cramps, 120, 121
Leg fracture, 128
Legg-Calvé-Perthes disease, 84
Leopold maneuvers, 224
Leukemia, 19, 51, 177, 180, 207, 210
Leukopenia, 180
Level of consciousness, 36, 108
levodopa (Dopar), 61, 158, 186
levothyroxine (Synthroid), 130, 217, 218
lidocaine (Xylocaine), 5, 32
Lightening, 147

Linea alba, 154
Linea nigra, 35, 154
Lipoproteins, 69, 159
Liquid diet, 136, 142
Listening, 172, 225
lithium
    effectiveness of, 222
    monitoring levels of, 4, 65
    salt intake and, 65
    therapeutic level of, 26, 218
lithium toxicity, 5, 38, 48, 65, 158, 188, 218
Lithotripsy, 221
Liver biopsy, 132, 220
Liver dysfunction, 92, 173, 217
Liver laceration or rupture, 62
Living will, 70
Lochia alba, rubra, and serosa, 58
Locked-in syndrome, 95
Logan bar, 73
Logrolling, 37
Lordosis, 177
Low-residue diet, 62, 141
Low-sodium diet, 78, 118
Lumbar puncture, 58
Lymphedema, 35, 44, 211
Lymphocyte count, 215

M

Magnesium, 113
    sources of, 176, 188, 201
magnesium sulfate, 46, 151, 169, 202
Magnetic resonance imaging, 167, 182
Malabsorption, 51
Malaise, 117
Malignant hyperthermia, 189
Malignant tumors, 174
Malpractice, 112
Mammography, 70
Manipulative behavior, 65, 216
mannitol (Osmitrol), 61, 88, 183

Maple syrup urine disease, 38
Maslow's hierarchy of needs, 3, 48
Mastectomy, 42, 44, 85, 208, 211, 212
Masturbation, 66, 200
Maxillofacial surgery, 133, 134
McBurney's sign, 22
McDonald's sign, 97
Mean arterial pressure, 153
Measles, 12, 69
Measurement systems, 104
Mechanical ventilation, 41, 102, 161, 169, 207, 210
Meconium, 147, 156
Mediastinum, 114
Medication administration, 71, 73, 80, 104, 107, 143, 168
Medulla oblongata, 108
Medulloblastoma, 21
Melanoma, 211
Melasma, 154
Menarche, 98
Ménière's disease, 170, 184
Meningitis, 49, 142, 166, 175, 183, 186
Meningomyelocele, 186
Menstruation, 98
Mental retardation, 98
meperidine (Demerol), 122, 221
Metabolic acidosis, 13, 56, 137, 143, 176, 195, 222
Metabolic alkalosis, 13, 138, 176, 213
Metabolism, 24
Metastasis, 90
methadone withdrawal in neonate, 17
Methergine, 202
methohexital (Brevital), 64
methylergonovine (Methergine), 75
methylphenidate (Ritalin), 65
methylprednisolone (Solu-Medrol), 92

Methylxanthine agents, 150
metronidazole (Flagyl), 49, 203, 204
Metrorrhagia, 61
miconazole (Monistat), 183
Migraine headache, 61
Milia, 98
Milk, 192, 196
Milwaukee brace, 47
Mineral oil, 102
Minnesota Multiphasic Personality Inventory, 95
Miotics, 10, 182
Mist tent (Croupette), 20, 23, 42, 186
Mitosis, 88
Mitral valve stenosis, 52
Modeling as behavior, 200
Molding of fetal head, 92
Monckeberg's sclerosis, 161
Mongolian spots, 148
Monoamine oxidase inhibitors, 14, 159, 219
Mononucleosis, 110
Moro's reflex, 11
morphine (Duramorph), 50, 54, 99, 226
Motor development, 19, 20
Multipara, 138
Multiple myeloma, 191
Multiple pregnancy, 155
Multiple sclerosis, 57, 61, 166, 186
Muscle pain, 85
Muscle relaxant, 195
Myasthenia gravis, 113, 145, 176, 177, 184
Mycoses, 131
Mydriatics, 109
Myelography, 16, 99
Myocardial infarction, 5, 18, 41, 50, 51, 77, 89, 111, 114, 115, 141, 163, 164, 195, 198, 199
Myometrium, 155
Myopia, 99
Myringotomy, 188
Myxedema coma, 126

N
Nägele's rule, 12
naloxone (Narcan), 68, 172, 210
Narcolepsy, 172
Narcotic abstinence syndrome, 63
Narcotic withdrawal in neonate, 17
Nasal fracture, 87
Nasogastric suctioning, 92
Nasogastric tube, 44, 51, 142, 151, 215
Nasotracheal suctioning, 26, 111, 215
Nausea, 122, 221
NCLEX examination, 199, 200
Nearsightedness, 126, 156
Neck dissection, 95, 210, 212
Neonatal period, 47
Neonate. See also Premature neonate.
  abnormal findings in, 147
  acquired immunodeficiency syndrome and, 53
  birth weight and, 76, 134, 147, 204, 210
  caloric intake of, 86
  cold stress and, 154
  establishing airway in, 47
  extramural birth and, 212
  head and chest circumference in, 46, 147
  hemoglobin level in, 134
  hyperinsulinism in, 91
  hypoglycemia in, 83
  immunization and, 39
  low-birth-weight, 34
  maintaining body temperature in, 147
  maintaining skin temperature of, 54
  period of reactivity in, 46
  positioning, 146, 213
  postmature, 69
  preventing blindness in, 50, 14, 2012

Neonate *(continued)*
   preventing heat loss in, 146, 183
   respiratory count in, 17
   respiratory depression in, 68
   skin creases in, 27
   suctioning, 146
   urine specific gravity in, 47
   vital signs of, 147
   vitamin K and, 16
   water percentage in body of, 23
   withdrawal in, 17, 18, 42
Nephrotic syndrome, 82, 190
Neural tube defects, 203
Neurogenic bladder, 72
Neuropathy, 214, 218
Neurosyphilis, 93
Nevus flammeus, 148
nifedipine (Procardia), 132, 162
Nitrazine paper, 73
Nitrogen balance, 209
nitroglycerin, 41, 50, 71, 108, 110, 113, 162, 169, 193
nitroprusside (Nitropress), 112, 152
Noncompliance, 97, 205
Nonmaleficence, 199
Nonstress test, 29
Nose blowing, 67
Nosocomial infection, 117
Nurse-patient relationship, 27-28, 111, 141, 157, 168. *See also* Trust.
Nurse's responsibilities, 101, 112, 116, 142
Nursing care plan, 116
Nursing diagnosis, 16, 103, 116, 166, 170, 171
Nursing process, 15
Nutrients, digestive process of, 69, 213
Nystagmus, 99

O
Obesity, 191, 222

Obsessive-compulsive disorder, 140, 218, 220
Obstipation, 62
On-call medication, 8
Ophthalmia neonatorum, 142, 213
Ophthalmic ointments, instilling, 39
Opiate withdrawal, 72
Opioids, 178, 226
Opportunistic infections, 18
Optic disk, 99
Oral care, 22
Orchitis, 22, 37, 150
Organic brain disorder, 63, 64, 97, 138
Organogenesis, 26
Orthopnea, 118, 211
Ortolani's sign, 38
Osmolarity, 176
Osteoarthritis, 112
Osteomyelitis, 119, 185
Osteoporosis, 70, 178, 225
Otitis externa, 205
Otitis media, 49, 57
Ovulation, 12, 93
Oxygen, arterial, partial pressure of, 14, 114
Oxygen saturation of venous blood, 160
Oxygen therapy, 50, 59, 87, 134, 150, 195, 201
oxytocin (Pitocin), 83, 87, 92, 119, 212

P
Pacemaker, 33, 77, 207, 211
Paget's disease, 188
Pain. *See also specific type.*
   administering medication for, 20
   blocking, 216
   chronic, 157
   distraction and, 204
   duration of, 204
   gate-control theory of, 173, 204
   interpreting, 74, 216
   intractable, 8
   postoperative, 141
   referred, 204

Pain *(continued)*
   signs of, 32, 202
   threshold of, 203
   tolerance of, 226
Palliative treatment, 111, 174
Palpitation, 74
Pancreas, exocrine function of, 6
Pancreatic cancer, 90, 212
Pancreatic enzyme replacement, 196
Pancreatitis, 57, 62, 94, 143, 186, 218, 219, 221, 222
pancrelipase (Pancrease), 115
Pancytopenia, 212
Para as number of pregnancies, 27
Paranoid personality disorder, 89, 218
Paraphimosis, 215
Paraphrasing as listening technique, 139
Parity, 154
Parkinson's disease, 36, 60-61, 117, 177, 184
paroxetine (Paxil), 110
Paroxysmal nocturnal dyspnea, 17, 165
Patient
   bathing, 129-130
   bed changes and, 64
   dying, 45
   false assurance to, 73
   health records and, 116
   lifting and moving, 63, 77, 172, 215
   repositioning, 107
   safety of, 3
Patient advocacy, 205
Patient-controlled analgesia, 172, 196, 216
Patient goals, 99, 138, 166
Patient's Bill of Rights, 71, 224
Patient self-determination, 107
Patient teaching, 172, 180
Pediatric dose calculation, 7

Pel-Ebstein fever, 25
Pelvic examination, 91, 169
Pelvic inflammatory disease, 38, 188, 189
Pelvic inlet, 46
Pelvic measurements, delivery and, 59
Pelvic-tilt exercises, 224
pemoline (Cylert), 220
penicillin, 80, 84, 113, 137, 148, 182
Penicillinase, 136
Peptic ulcer, 17, 18, 84. *See also* Gastric ulcer.
Percussion as assessment technique, 99, 105
Percutaneous transluminal coronary angioplasty, 161
Pericardiocentesis, 57
Pericarditis, 33, 159, 164
Peritoneal dialysis, 21, 39, 57, 95, 152
permethrin (Nix) shampoo, 185
Pernicious anemia, 2, 149, 173, 210, 214
PERRLA, 107
Personality disorder, 216. *See also specific type.*
Petechiae, 25, 225
Phantom limb pain, 123
Pharmacology, 144
Pharyngitis, 182
phenazopyridine (Pyridium), 100
Phenothiazine derivative, 158
phenylephrine (Neo-Synephrine), 22
Phenylketonuria, 20, 143, 146, 149, 219
phenytoin (Dilantin), 35, 65, 186, 219
Pheochromocytoma, 182
Phimosis, 137
Phobic disorder, 4, 26, 177, 218
Phosphate sources, 225
Phototherapy, 67, 212
Physical examination, 103

Physical therapy, 63
Pica, 92
Pilocarpine, 182
Pituitary gland, 145
Placenta, 75
Placenta previa, 37, 42, 47, 74, 206
Planning as nursing process step, 16
Platelets, 151
Play therapy, 99
Pleasure principle, 68
Pleural friction rub, 197
Pleurisy, 67
Pleuritis, 13
Pneumatic antishock garment, 81
Pneumocystis carinii pneumonia, 101, 210
Pneumomeningitis, 166
Pneumonectomy, 100, 208
Pneumonia, 118, 207
Pneumothorax, 17, 101
Point of maximal impulse, 118
Poison, ingested, 43, 45, 141, 186, 191
Polio vaccine, 94
Polycythemia vera, 10, 151
Polydactyly, 147
Polyuria, 13
Pons, 98
Portals of exit, substances expelled through, 87
Portal hypertension, 117, 219, 223
Port-wine stain, 148
Positive end-expiratory pressure, 201
Positron emission tomography, 98
Postanesthesia care unit, 8, 31, 38, 173-174
Postmortem care, 123, 141
Postoperative complications, 32, 105, 111, 129, 143, 173, 174, 178, 183, 184, 202, 220
Postoperative events, teaching child about, 31
Postoperative patient, 68

Postoperative period, vital signs in, 9
Postpartum bleeding, 60, 75, 207
Postpartum depression, 141
Postpartum patient, 67, 119
Posttraumatic stress disorder, 177, 223
Postural drainage, 3, 107. *See also* Chest physiotherapy.
Potassium, 30, 95, 215
sources of, 118, 142, 201
potassium chloride, 13
Potassium supplements, 215
Practical nurse's responsibilities, 109
prednisone (Deltasone), 86, 95
Preeclampsia. *See* Pregnancy-induced hypertension.
Pregnancy
acceptance of, 191
alcohol intake and, 14
ankle edema and, 150, 154
avoiding medications during, 93
caloric intake and, 121
complications of, 12, 152
diet recommendations for, 79
duration of, 131
ectopic, 27, 95
folic acid in, 92
F/TPAL system and, 154
hemodilution of, 153
infection transmission and, 119
iron supplements and, 122
nausea and vomiting in, 122
radiography and, 98
sexual activity and, 98
signs of, 12, 97, 98, 154
urine glucose in, 177

Pregnancy *(continued)*
  uterus length in, 59
  vaginal bleeding in, 47, 207
  vaginal examination and, 207
  venous return and, 150
  visualization in, 153
  vitamin therapy and, 79
  water intake during, 30
  weight gain during, 6, 73
Pregnancy-induced hypertension, 12, 28, 37, 42, 91, 138, 140, 157
Pregnancy risk categories for drugs, 94
Prejudice, 194
Premature neonate, 3, 19, 20, 27, 141, 197, 210, 211
Premature ventricular contractions, 5
Premenstrual syndrome, 85
Presbycusis, 226
Presbyopia, 22, 99
Prescriptions, 143
Pressure ulcers, 2, 40, 53, 61, 128, 135, 145, 226
Prevention, 206
probenecid (Benemid), 8, 165, 182
progesterone, 154
Projection in psychiatry, 75, 220
Prolactin, 6, 116
Prophylaxis, 111
propranolol (Inderal), 77, 162
Prostaglandin gel, 147
Prostate cancer, 22, 107, 169
Prostatectomy, 24, 53, 178
Prostate-specific antigen, 22
Prostate surgery, 121
Prostatitis, 23
protamine sulfate, 52, 140, 202
Protein, 117

Protein-calorie malnutrition, 48
Protein systemic shunt, 187
Prothrombin, 57
Protocols, 116
Psychiatric patient, 48, 191, 195, 218
Psychoanalytic theory, 66
Psychodrama, 48
Psychotropic medications, 64, 65, 66, 217
Ptosis, 40
Pulmonary artery catheterization, 160
Pulmonary artery pressure, 25, 160
Pulmonary artery pressure catheter, 159
Pulmonary artery wedge pressure, 25, 160
Pulmonary edema, 5, 18, 90, 92, 159, 165
Pulmonary embolism, 14, 73, 100, 119, 133, 159, 191, 212
Pulmonary function tests, 132
Pulse amplitude and rhythm, 31
Pulse deficit, 3
Pulse pressure, widening, 11
Pulse rate, 13, 32, 78, 103, 106, 108, 110
Pulsus alternans, 81
Pulsus paradoxus, 86
Pureed diet, 136
Purple glove syndrome, 65
Purpura, 25
Pursed-lip breathing, 21, 149
Pyelography, 215
Pyloric stenosis, 51
pyridostigmine (Mestinon), 113

Q
Quality assurance, 71
Quickening, 12

R
Rabies, 30
RACE acronym, 10
Radiant warmer, 54, 146
Radiation therapy, 55, 112, 117, 224
Radioactive implant, 55, 60, 120, 174-175, 178
Radioactivity, exposure to, 123
Radiography, 98
Range-of-motion exercises, 108, 135, 173, 176
Rapid-eye-movement sleep, 172
Raynaud's disease, 105
Raynaud's phenomenon, 96, 105
Reaction formation in psychiatry, 76
Rectal tube, 63, 89
Red blood cells, 35, 79
Red cell indices, 114
Red reflex, 191
Reflexes, grading, 67
Refraction, 126
Reframing as therapeutic technique, 99
Refusal of treatment, 115
Regression to earlier stage, 76
Reiter's syndrome, 146
Relaxin, 154
Religious customs, 177, 203, 205, 206, 226
Renal biopsy, 82
Renal calculi, 103, 141
Renal disease, 153, 222
Renal failure, 10, 12, 221, 222
Renal trauma, 188
Repression as defense mechanism, 75, 220
Required surgery, 73
Resistance exercises, 135, 173
Respirations, counting, 78, 108
Respiratory acidosis, 13, 137, 176, 211

Respiratory alkalosis, 13, 102, 137, 176
Respiratory complications, 183
Respiratory depression, 31, 68, 189
Respiratory distress, 19, 50, 142, 202, 210
Respiratory distress syndrome, 20, 67, 68, 119
Respiratory failure, 179, 209
Respiratory paralysis, 66
Respiratory tract infections, 134
Restraints, 18, 20, 28, 42, 64, 130, 131, 172
Retention enema, 177
Retinal detachment, 127, 137, 185, 189
Retinopathy, 204
Reverse isolation, 52
Reye's syndrome, 95
Rheumatic fever, 140, 151, 182, 185, 194
Rheumatoid arthritis, 26, 55, 85
Rh$_O$(D) immune globulin (RhoGAM), 121
Rhonchi, 3, 178, 197
Rinne test, 100
ritodrine (Yutopar), 151
Rocky Mountain spotted fever, 33, 168, 183, 187
Romberg test, 190, 204
Rooting reflex, 148, 208
Rubella, 7, 9, 122, 212
Rule of Nines, 107
Rule utilitarianism, 200

S
Safer sexual practices, 70
Salicylates, 85
Salicylate toxicity. See aspirin toxicity.
Salivation, 76
Salmonellosis, 188
Sarcoma, 63
Scalp vein infusion, 34
Scarlet fever, 187

Schick test, 58
Schizophrenia, 48, 216
Scoliosis, 38, 47, 187
scopolamine transdermal patch (Transderm-Scop), 150
Scrotal edema, 150
Scrotal examination, 137
Scurvy, 133
Sebaceous glands, 225
Seclusion in psychiatry, 14
Seizures, 35, 36, 61, 168, 183
Semilunar valves, 104
Sengstaken-Blakemore tube, 6
Sensory deprivation, 170
Sensory loss, 190
Sensory overload, 170
Separation anxiety, 191
Septicemia, 33
Septic shock, 82, 184
Sequela, 74
Seroconversion, 179
Serotonin reuptake inhibitors, 110
sertraline (Zoloft), 110
Setting-sun sign, 56
Sexual assault, 61, 119
Sexual intercourse, 110, 119, 120, 164
Sheehan's syndrome, 97
Shingles. See Herpes zoster.
Shock, 3, 15, 123
Sickle cell anemia, 8, 25, 40, 67, 150, 193, 209
Sickle cell crisis, 74, 89, 193, 209
Sigmoidoscopy, 44
Sinoatrial node, 114
Sitz bath, 170
Sjögren's syndrome, 175
Skeletal traction, 59, 189, 193
Skin graft, 74, 168, 178, 184, 189
Skin preparation for injection, 144
Skull fracture, 222
Skull X-ray, 64
Sleep aids, 171, 214, 215
Sleep apnea, 171

Sleep cycle, 88
Sodium, 95, 123
sodium polystyrene sulfonate enema, 109
Soft diet, 136
Somnambulism, 62, 172
Sore throat, 87
Speech impediment, 171
Spermatozoa, 110
Sperm count, 97, 206
Spica cast, 29
Spinal anesthesia, 38
Spinal block, 92
Spinal cord injury, 81, 92, 93, 166, 186, 196
Spinal fusion, 37
Spinal shock, 57, 81
Sprains, 99
Sputum culture, 167
Sputum specimen, 58, 131, 132
Standard precautions, 28, 30, 90, 96, 131, 172
Standards of care, 69
Standing orders, 116
Starling's law, 115
Status epilepticus, 36, 56, 168, 187
Sterile field, maintaining, 126, 173
Steroid therapy, 19, 85-86, 179, 211
Stethoscope, 39, 94
Stillbirth, 91
Stoma care, 109, 143
Stomal retraction, 48
Stomatitis, 57, 211
Stool color, 64
Stool specimens, 62, 131
Stork bites, 121
Strabismus, 117
Strains, 99
Streptococcal infections, 117
Streptomycin, 185
Stress incontinence, 103
Stress management, 64, 173
Stroke, 21, 88, 93, 98, 127, 128, 176
Stroke volume, 81, 164
Stye, 137

Subcutaneous injection, 108, 143
Subinvolution, 212
Sublimation in psychiatry, 75
Subluxation, 63
Substance abuse, 122
sucralfate (Carafate), 58
Suicide, 26, 34, 196, 202, 218
Sundowner syndrome, 172
Superego, 12
Supine hypotensive syndrome, 150, 154, 195
Suppression of thoughts, 47
Suppressor T cells, 95
Surgery, preparation for, 32, 122, 173, 184
Swan-Ganz catheter, 159
Sweat test, 60
Syphilis, 23, 38, 50, 123, 127
Systemic lupus erythematosus, 26, 56, 187

T
tamoxifen (Nolvadex), 169, 207
Tantrums, 194
Tardive dyskinesia, 151, 219
Tay-Sachs disease, 146
Teenage pregnancy, 34
Teeth, 107
Telangiectatic nevi, 121
Telephone orders, 115
Tensilon test, 176
terbutaline (Brethine), 151
Testicular self-examination, 71
Testicular surgery, 206
Tetanus, 101
Tetany, 24
tetracycline, 112, 150, 158, 187
Tetralogy of Fallot, 111, 137, 189
Thalassemia, 71
theophylline (Theo-Dur), 150, 211

theophylline toxicity, 42
Therapeutic relationship, 66, 195-196
Thiamine deficiency, 214
thiopental (Pentothal), 109
Third-party payer, 168, 201
Third spacing of fluid, 157
Thoracentesis, 101, 209
Thought blocking, 24
Thought broadcasting, 158
thrombin, 117
Thrombocytopenia, 122, 180
Thromboembolism, 128
Thrombophlebitis, 24, 44, 109, 134, 210
Thrombus formation, 225
Thrush. See Candidiasis.
Thyroid deficiency, 193
Thyroidectomy, 79, 85, 217, 219, 220, 222
Thyroid replacement therapy, 83, 217
Thyroid storm, 151
Tilt table, 40
Timed-release medication, 108
Tinea infection, 184
Tocolytic therapy, 90, 151
Toddler, 47, 188, 195
Toilet training, 50, 75, 196
tolbutamide (Orinase), 120
Tolerance of drug, 28
Tonometry, 132
Tonsillectomy, 54
TORCH infections, 96
Total parenteral nutrition, 23, 38, 56, 59, 81
Tourniquets, rotating, 84
Toxic shock syndrome, 17, 81, 205
Toxoplasmosis, 121
Tracheal suction, 102
Tracheobronchial suctioning, 17
Tracheostomy care, 29, 62, 107, 108, 224
Trajectory nursing, 203, 216

Transcutaneous electrical nerve stimulation, 203
Transfer techniques, 39, 40, 108
Transfusion reactions, 30, 57, 81, 169, 202
Transient ischemic attacks, 22, 176, 211
Transplantation, immunosuppressant therapy and, 37
Transplant rejection, 41, 68, 221
Transurethral resection of the prostate, 37
Transvestism, 219
Trauma patient, 44, 94, 143, 188
Treadmill test, 114
Trendelenburg test, 123
Trichomoniasis, 82, 204, 226
Tricyclic antidepressants, 90, 191, 192
trihexyphenidyl (Artane), 219
Trismus, 101
Trousseau's sign, 6
Trust, 193, 195, 225. See also Nurse-patient relationship.
T tube, 170, 174, 184
Tube feeding, 56, 83, 122
Tuberculin skin test, 6, 30, 140
Tuberculosis, 6, 59, 97, 171, 209
Tumors, 181, 212. See also specific type.
Tzanck test, 167

U
Ulcerative colitis, 70, 186, 187
Umbilical blood sampling, 155
Umbilical cord, 9, 27, 34, 146, 192
Underwater exercise as therapy, 82
Upper respiratory tract, 83

Urea, 226
Urethral calculi, 141
Urge incontinence, 104
Urgent surgery, 73
Urinary frequency, 10
Urinary incontinence, 10
Urinary tract infections, 24, 70, 79, 117, 165, 213, 214, 223
Urine acidification, 165
Urine culture, 20
Urine incontinence, 104. *See also specific type.*
Urine output, 15, 156, 208
Urine pH, 82
Urine, residual, 15, 213
Urine specific gravity, 47, 87
Urine specimen, 58, 73, 88, 128, 182, 211, 214
Urine volume, 112
Urticaria, 57
Uterine atony, 155, 207
Uterine contractions, 13, 14, 15, 57, 76, 98, 155, 202
Uterus, massaging, 67, 210
Utilization review, 201

V

Vaginal bleeding, 47, 207, 208
Vaginal infection, 120, 168, 183, 203, 204
Vagotomy, 4
Valsalva's maneuver, 4
Value cohort, 201
Values clarification, 224
Valvular insufficiency, 52
Varicose veins, 115, 140
Vascular resistance, 123
Vasectomy, 150, 224
Vegetarian diet, 107, 213
Venipuncture, 40, 55
Venous blood, 80
Venous stasis, 134
Venous stasis ulcer, 127
Venous thrombosis, 109
Ventilators, 41, 75. *See also* Mechanical ventilation.

Ventricular septal defect, 77
Veracity, 199
verapamil (Calan, Isoptin), 89, 111, 162
Verbal orders, 115
Vernix caseosa, 148
Vertigo, 67, 170
vincristine (Oncovin), 169, 207
Visual acuity, 22, 80
Vital organ perfusion, 5
Vitamin, 133
Vitamin B complex, 31
Vitamin B_6, 101
Vitamin B_{12}, 86
Vitamin B_{12} supplements, 107
Vitamin C, 117, 215
Vitamin C deficiency, 14
Vitamin D, foods high in, 91
Vitamin K, 16, 28
Vitiligo, 138
Voiding after surgery, 61
Vomiting, 110, 122, 221
Von Willebrand's disease, 25

W

Walker use, 177
warfarin (Coumadin), 158
Wasting syndrome, 18
Water-hammer pulse, 159
Weber's test, 100
Weight, measuring, 31
Weight loss, 215
Wheezing, 67, 178, 183, 197
White blood cell differential, 114
Wilms' tumor, 122, 202
Wisdom teeth, 68
Wound care, 167
Wound healing, 117, 145, 165
Wristdrop, 8

XYZ

Young's rule, pediatric dose calculation and, 7

zidovudine (Retrovir), 55, 179
Zoster immune globulin, 165
Z-track I.M. injection, 9, 35, 197